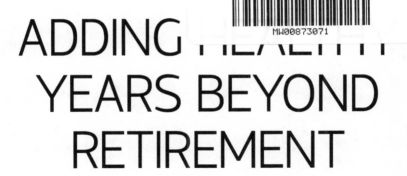

ADDING HEALTHY YEARS BEYOND RETIREMENT

DR. RAMACHANDRA HEGDE
BHANDIMANE

Dedicated to supercentenarian and a great humanitarian, His Holiness Padma Bhushan Dr. Shivakumar Swamiji, the pontiff (April 1, 1907- January 21, 2019) of Sri Siddaganga Mutt, Tumakuru, Karnataka, India

Contents

Disclaimer

This book is not a substitute for consulting physician.Neither the author nor the publisher shall be liable for any loss arising from any suggestion in this book

Prologue

Why this book on retirement?

We cannot avoid retirement and old age. As the age advances the hair turns grey, hair falls from the head; skin shows the signs of wrinkles, power of eyesight and ear reduces. These are everyday things. Whatever cosmetics and body conditioners we use to mask the age, a day will sure to come we will be exposed. So accepting the reality is the best choice.

I am always surprised to hear the conversation among my senior colleagues about health, family, and retirement. Much before their actual retirement, many people have gone into depression, fearing that they will soon lose power, position, and respect in life at home and in society. Thinking more about career, children, family and social life, economic insecurity etc. people get many modern lifestyle-related non-communicable diseases like hypertension (HTN), cardiovascular diseases (CVDs), brain stroke, diabetes, asthma, cancer, dementia, anxiety, depression and bipolar disorder, disturbed sleep, bone and nerve disorders. Though I also faced some problems of the types mentioned above, it was never so acute as to need regular medication. Hence, I decided that I would continue to be mentally occupied even after retirement without a break since fitness should be the top priority. It may not be for money but a respectable occupation so that there is no time to think about body aches or headaches.

After retirement at 60, fortunately, I got a full-time work opportunity one after another in four organizations in new roles unrelated to my previous profession. Over time, one of my former colleagues suggested that I author a book based on my experience so that people get motivated to work after retirement and get a new lease of life free from diseases. This book is based on some assumptions to lead a peaceful life viz. "Work is Worship, Work is Wealth, Work is Health and Health is Heaven"; "All Good Deeds

Lead to God"; "Life journey should be on the path of truth and honesty"; "Life is a Challenge-Face it, Life is Game-Play it, Life is a Dream-Realize it"; "All people around us are good".

I attended several farewell functions and every event is a replica of one another. The youngsters bring the shower of praises, and the retirees say that they have completed long years of hard work and stressful life. Now they will take a break as they have plenty of time for reading newspapers, watching TV, walking in the company of retired people etc. Some people said they would think over after six months or a year or so what to do. However, I noticed such people never started at all.

The primary purpose of bringing out this non-medical book is to provide various parameters which can contribute to health, happiness and longevity. While compiling, I could visit multiple websites and refer to many publications relevant to the topic appended in the reference chapter to get more information.

Possessing a healthy body and adding healthy years to one's life is everybody's dream. Despite advances in the medical sciences and technology people continue to suffer from one or the other form of ailment. I have tried to convey a holistic approach to have healthy ageing in this book. Nobody is eternal. But combining mental and physical activities and maintaining time and self-discipline for work, food, sleep, and exercise can postpone the morbidity issue and keep away from the doctor. The twelve chapters revolve around a common theme but exist independently. There is a saying "Getting old is mandatory but feeling old is optional". There is no fitness formula for one's wellbeing but one has to develop one by observing body reactions. Adding years to life is nothing but postponing the illness. Keeping busy schedule, adding new qualifications and experience, visiting new locations and meeting new people, trying to lead a stress-free life, considering every day as an adventure and a challenge contribute to good health. Important thing after retirement is that we should love whatever work we do. As most of the books on retirement speak on money multiplication plans, social security, savings and investments, medical insurance, tax planning, etc., I have not covered these topics.

I thank my wife, Parvati, for providing a proper environment at home. Thanks to youngsters my children Vani and Veena, nephew Vikas who read the manuscript and made suggestions for improvement. I also thank my classmate Dr Narayan Hegde, Managing Trustee, Nisargopachar Gram Sudhar Trust, Urulikanchan and formerly president BAIF, Pune, my former colleague Mr N.R.Kannan, Bengaluru, Ex- Chief General Manager, NABARD, and many friends volunteered to read the manuscript and give valuable suggestions. I am also indebted to many people with whom I discussed their experiences with ageing. I documented my own life experience referring many gerontology research studies to overcome old age gloom to lead a healthy life after retirement. I hope this book will be helpful to one and all.

Ramachandra Hegde Bhandimane

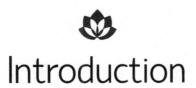

Introduction

Retirement is one of the most critical crossroads one faces when one stops regularly working from nine to five or ten to six jobs. It involves a fundamental change in lifestyle that calls for a new outlook on how we approach each day. It will generally occur when a person reaches the age bracket of 60-65 years. Ideally, they cannot earn further their regular income, but they can live life on their terms. The retired people face one or the other multiple problems like loneliness, financial difficulties, poor health, the lower status of power, poor sleep, less physical activity, bladder and bowel issues, history of falling, visual and hearing impairments, chronic pain and frailty

However, some people never retire and face none of the above old age problems. For instance, a) Dr. John B Goodenough (b. July 25, 1922) is German-American Professor and solid-state physicist. He is currently 100 years old but still works as a mechanical engineering and material science professor at the University of Texas at Austin. Dr. John B Goodenough won the 2019 Nobel Prize for chemistry for developing lithium rechargeable batteries. He shared the prize with British-American chemist M. Stanley Whittingham and a Japanese chemist Yoshino Akira. b) Dr. Shigeaki Hinohara (October 4, 1911- July 18, 2017) was a Japanese physician who died at 105. He continued to see patients until a month before his death and frequently offered advice on living well. Described by his colleagues as Japan's national treasure, he headed five foundations and was president of St. Lukes International Hospital in Tokyo. The secrets of Dr.

Hinohara's longevity is given under the chapter the spirit of living later in this book. c) Wikipedia reveals a list of about 40 centenarian medical professionals who continued to work beyond 100.

We are all aware that impermanence is the only reality-the truth. Everyone born on the planet has to leave one day. The idea is not to prolong one's life but to lead a healthy life as long as we destined to live and to be happy and valuable. It is in our own hands to a large extent. We create our health and destiny! Who does not want to live long and live well? Retirement, ageing and death are inevitable for everyone. Every birthday reminds us that we are nearer to the end by one year. We should accept that the body degenerates, and one has to leave this world or body flesh. Retirement is a dread word due to the fear of losing power and position that no one will care for them. But in fact, post-retirement leads them to become masters of their own time to choose their own pace and activities. However, one should develop a sense of purpose for work, social life and meaningful interaction to keep busy from dawn to dusk to enjoy a healthy, happy and peaceful life. One should remember that retirement pertains only to the organisation's work but does not apply to life. Retiring is giving up that old identity and re-inventing a new role such as babysitter for the grandchildren, home maker, volunteer for social work, and anything with a sense of purpose without stress. New engagement can be reading, writing, meditation, self-study, which brings happiness which is nothing but a spiritual experience with love, grace and gratitude.

What are the different names for age?

Though everybody wants to stay young and vital throughout life, ageing surrounds by many myths and questions. While old age signs appear for the body, the mind could always be as young as a child. Gerontology researchers have given the age several names, say chronological age, biological age, social age, subjective age, personal age (feel-age, look-age, do-age, and interest age), cognitive age etc. But for discussion, it is restricted to three categories viz. chronological (number age), biological (physiological) and psychological (mental). The first is calculated based on one's date of birth; the health conditions determine the second, and the third is how old one feels at heart. Though one cannot control the first, one can take care of their second with good diet, physical activities, and a positive attitude. Positive thinking and optimism can reverse the cognitive age, which refers to memory, learning and self-esteem. Chronological and physiological ages do not always coincide, and physical appearance and health status often do not always correspond to typical at a particular chronological age. Similarly, a recorded person could be psychologically young.

What is happening to our brains as age advances?

We feel less sharp or slower to process information. Doctors have traditionally found it difficult to assess the rate at which our brains are ageing. For some, these changes will come early, and for some, they will go lately. Some people even have genetics that protects them from having virtually any changes at all. What seems to work even better is having a fit body. Research shows that being physically fit will help keep our brains in good shape, too. Even just moderate walking for 30 minutes a day has been shown to help reduce the ageing brain's rate shrink. And the idea that what we eat applies to our brain as well as our body.

All humans and other living organisms change with time. As a multidimensional reality of life, ageing is difficult to define. The National Institute on Ageing (NIA) is one of the 27 Institutes and Centers of the National Institute of Health (NIH), which leads a broad scientific effort to understand the nature of ageing and extend the healthy and active years of life. NIA is the primary US Federal agency headquartered in Baltimore, the USA, supporting and conducting research on Alzheimer's disease. It states that "in its broadest sense, ageing merely refers to degenerating changes that occur during the lifespan".

Remain Fit-Key to Happiness:

"Fitness First" should be the goal after retirement. Because if we fall sick, it will bring problem not only for us but also for our kith and kin. Fitness means physical and mental, spiritual, and psychological because all these factors constitute an individual's health, happiness, and longevity. Good health is also a mystery because there are people after 60 even up to 100, very fit to undertake everyday activities with vigour and vitality. At the same time, some die at an early age despite having access to best medical facilities. The research studies reveal those who are workaholic, social and volunteers for community service live long without facing significant health issues.

I believe that "age is just a number" means that a person's chronological age does not necessarily reflect how they act. There are many sexagenarians (60-69), septuagenarians (70-79), octogenarians(80-89), non agenarians(90-99) and centenarians(100-109) who are very active, both mentally and physically, and others in their thirties who seem old due to their attitudes and way of living. There is no uniform fitness formula for everyone. As fingerprints of anyone do not match with any other in the world, similarly, the fitness formula recommended for one does not hold good for another one.

Usually, people set milestones in their lives such as education, careers, marriage, owning a house or a car, getting children, and then thinking about their future. If we believe life is a gift meant to enjoy the fullest, it will always be beautiful. An ageing study by Purdue University revealed that one is old as one feels. The research team interviewed about 500 people between the ages of 55 and 74 between 1995 and 2005. At the study's outset, the results indicated that most of these folks felt about 12 years younger than their chronological age. Schafer writes that people feel younger because of the extreme emphasis on being youthful in today's culture. "People want to feel younger, and so when they consider inevitable chronological age, they can lose a lot of confidence in their cognitive abilities." Studies have proved that people who do not follow a healthy lifestyle and pessimists are more likely to suffer a range of illnesses from aches and pains to high blood pressure and die younger than their optimistic counterparts.[1]

Biological age also called physiological age, measures how well or poorly our body functions relative to our actual calendar age. For example, we may have a chronological age of 65. Still, because of a healthy and active lifestyle (free from longevity threats like tobacco and obesity), our body is physiologically more similar to someone with a chronological age of 55. Our biological age would, therefore, be 55.

Factors That Determine Biological Age

There are several ways to determine one's biological age, but none are definitive or accurate. However, there are health factors that would give us years back on our average life expectancy. Healthy lifestyle habits can significantly impact our longevity and biological age, including exercise habits, eating habits, stress levels, alcohol consumption, level of education, and amount of sleep. Another major contributor to biological age is heredity or our gene pool. Just as specific diseases run in families, longevity also does. If we have family members who have lived longer than 96 years, the chances are that we will also live a long life, even if our habits are less than healthy. Another essential factor influencing biological age is where we live. It is no secret that the environment and culture we live in connect to healthy habits.[2, 3]

Our Chronological Age is Different from Our Biological Age:

A ground-breaking study confirmed that people age at different rates. Our biological age can reveal a great deal about our general health and the rate we are ageing. This study was unique in that it did not focus its ageing research on older subjects. Instead, the scientists' objective was to reveal more about the ageing process in younger people, and therefore provide a foundation for devising preventative therapies for age-related diseases.

A cohort of nearly 1,000 participants born in New Zealand in 1972 and 1973 underwent extensive testing at ages 26, 32, and 38. These tests measured 18 different biological markers that each forms a piece of the ageing puzzle. Each participant's health concerning pulmonary, periodontal, cardiovascular, renal, hepatic, and immune systems was assessed using these biomarkers. With these results, researchers calculated a biological age for each participant and then compared the changes in these measurements over time, yielding a quantified pace of ageing. The majority of the participants had biological ages similar to their chronological age. Still, some participants were found to have aged as much as three years physiologically for only one calendar year. Furthermore, scientists found that participants with an accelerated rate of ageing performed worse on physical and cognitive ability assessments.

The common saying, "We are as old (or young) as we feel," also came true in this study. Participants with an older biological age perceived themselves to be in poorer health than their biologically younger peers. And in case we need even more convincing to take better care of ourselves, independent observers scored participants with higher biological ages as looking older than their biologically younger peers as well though all of the participants were the same age chronologically.

One of the biggest challenges in assessing ageing is that it is essentially caused by all of the cumulative experiences we have throughout our lives. For doctors and scientists, it is nearly impossible to determine whether lifestyle, stress, medical history, or other circumstances are individually responsible for many age-related diseases. Ultimately, it is a combination of all these factors that either ages us prematurely or keeps us healthy and prevents illnesses. This is precisely why so many biomarkers were used in the study and why multiple beneficial lifestyle choices typically synergistically affect our overall health.

This study will have significant implications on further research to prevent ageing, which will help us not only increase our lifespan, but more importantly, increase our healthspan, or "the years of life lived without disease and disability." Living longer doesn't help us much if we are too sick to enjoy the extra years we have fully. Making proactive decisions about your health now can have lasting positive effects.

Biomarkers of ageing would give the proper "biological age", which may differ from the chronological age. Although greying of hair increases with age, hair greying cannot be called a biomarker of ageing. Similarly, skin wrinkles and other expected changes seen with ageing are not better indicators of future functionality than chronological age. Bio-gerontologists have continued efforts to find and validate biomarkers of ageing, but success thus far has been limited.

Our calendar age determines the date we were born. Although we consider this chronological age our actual age, we often overlook that some people with a recorded age of 50 may be as fit as 30-year-olds. Yet, others have a chronological age of 35, but their physical condition is 60 years old. To determine a person's actual state of health, we must examine their biological age. Biological age is calculated based on a person's physical and mental condition - and therefore expresses their true age.[4]

Possessing a healthy body and adding healthy years to one's life is everybody's cherished dream. But despite advances in medical science and technology, people suffer from various forms of diseases. The twentieth century was an era of acute infectious diseases, such as tuberculosis, smallpox, diphtheria, tetanus etc., and comprising 80% of all deaths in 1900. With these diseases nearly eradicated by the 1970s, mortality has been reduced by almost 99%. Still, in the twenty-first century, modern lifestyle-related non-communicable diseases like hypertension, cardiovascular diseases (CVDs), stroke, diabetes, asthma, cancer, dementia, anxiety, and depression are causing morbidity, affecting the ability of people to add healthy years to their lives.

One notable aspect of population ageing is the increase in the number of people who live to the age of 100. In 2009, there were an estimated 455,000 centenarians in the world. By 2050, their number is projected to rise to 4.1 million, a nine-fold increase.

Yet this gift for many can become a problem – because we have not imagined a new approach to a long life lived well. Ageing well requires a series of transitions that change where we live, how we live, and our roles and responsibilities in our communities.

The most common misperception on ageing is that the life after 60, the older one gets, the sicker and more disabled. In his study of centenarians, Dr. Thomas Perl argues instead for a more optimistic and enabling point of view, noting that "the older an individual gets, the healthier he or she has been." There is evidence to support his observation. The Gallup-Healthways Well-Being Index – a large sample size, continuing poll – has demonstrated that individuals over 65 consistently report higher degrees of overall wellbeing than any other age group. The polling data indicate that better eating habits, greater access to healthcare, and improved emotional health contribute to this group's high score, despite physical wellbeing declines.

The focus of healthcare needs to shift from treating illness to promoting wellness. Individuals who remain healthy and active as they age can stay productive and engaged in the community, which has profound implications for their wellbeing and their families, communities, and societies. Helping older persons to deal more effectively with personal transitions of ageing begins with effective and targeted health care and preventive services.

The world's most extensive study conducted during 2017-18 on the aged-the Longitudinal Ageing Study in India (LA-SI) reported that 75 million Indians above 60 suffer from chronic diseases. While 27 per cent of the elderly have multi-morbidities, around 40 per cent have one or another disability, and 20 per cent have issues related to mental health. The LASI, Wave1, covered a baseline sample of 72,250 individuals aged 45 and above and their spouses. This included 31,464 persons aged 60 and above and 6,749 persons aged 75 and above. In the 2011 census, the 60+ accounted for 8.6 per cent of India's population, accounting for 103 million older people. Growing at around 3 per cent annually, the number of elderly age population will rise to

319 million in 2050.

The survey used bio-markers based on direct health examinations to estimate the prevalence of chronic health conditions. Around three-quarters of those 60 and above who were diagnosed with chronic illnesses have been treated for hypertension (77%), heart diseases (74%), diabetes mellitus (83%), lung diseases (72%) and cancer (75%). More than half of the elderly have been treated for stroke (58%) and bone or joint diseases (56%), whereas the treatment rate for neurological, psychological, and psychiatric disorders is 41%.

Life expectancy varies widely throughout the world, from roughly 50 years in Sierra Leone to nearly 84 years in Japan. India's life expectancy is 68 years. The research studies also demonstrate that only 20 - 30% of life expectancy is genetic, whereas 70 - 80% of the variation is due to environment, behaviour and circumstance. Thus a vast majority of the factors influencing life expectancy are modifiable.

The World Happiness Report 2018 compares the survey data collected from 156 countries by their happiness levels. The research conducted from 2012 to 2016 asked people to assess their level of satisfaction with life on a scale of zero to ten. Finland is the happiest country globally, with Norway, Denmark, Iceland, and Switzerland holding the successive top positions. Sweden is not far standing at number 9. The US comes in at a modest number18. India figures close to the bottom at 133. It is disheartening to know that Pakistan (75), Bhutan (97), Nepal (101) and Bangladesh (115) are considerably higher than India on the chart. The factors considered to arrive for wellbeing are general health, mental health, income and employment. Scandinavian countries score high with their elaborate social safety nets, including free schools and hospitals, parental leave, generous unemployment benefits, and later life care for older people.[5]Ensuing chapters discuss critical factors for good health and longevity.

CHAPTER TWO

History of Retirement

Retirement, or the practice of leaving one's job or ceasing to work after reaching a certain age, has been around since the 18th century. Before the 18th century, the average life expectancy of people was between 26 and 40 years. Due to this, only a tiny percentage of the population reached an age where physical impairments became obstacles to working-work until you die - or until you can't work anymore. Until the late 19thcentury, that was the old-age plan for the bulk of the world's workers. If you were alive, you worked probably on a farm-or, if you were wealthier, managed a farm or more significant estate. When farming dominated the economy in the United States, most men worked as long as their health permitted. As they aged, though, they often cut their hours and turned the most physically demanding chores over to sons or hired hands. In 1880, when half of Americans worked on a farm, 78 per cent of American men worked past age 65.

Many people choose to retire when they are eligible for private or public pension benefits. However, some were forced to retire when physical conditions no longer allowed them to work (by illness or accident) or due to legislation concerning their position. In most countries, the idea of retirement is of recent origin, introduced during the late 19th and early 20th centuries. Previously, low life expectancy and the absence of pension arrangements meant that most workers continued to work until death. Germany was the first country to introduce retirement in 1889.

Nowadays, most developed countries have systems to provide pensions on retirement in old age, which employers or the state may sponsor. In many poorer countries, support for the aged is still mainly provided through the family. Today, retirement with a pension is considered a right of the worker in many societies. Intense ideological, social, cultural and political battles were fought over to consider pension as a right. In many western countries this right is mentioned in national constitutions. Retirement as a government policy began to be adopted by countries during the late 19th century and the 20th century, starting in Germany under Otto Von Bismarck.

The normal retirement age in selected countries is in brackets. United Kingdom(68), Germany, Greece, Italy, Netherlands, Norway, Spain, United States(67), Austria, Belgium, Denmark, France, Sweden, Switzerland(65), India, Thailand (60), and Cambodia (55) [Source: OECD]

The social security system and retirement-The German Precedent:

It is fascinating to know how retirement was invented. Germany became the first nation to adopt an old-age social insurance program in 1889, designed by Germany's Chancellor, Otto von Bismarck. At Bismarck's behest, the idea was first put forward in 1881 by Germany's Emperor, William the First, in a ground-breaking letter to the German Parliament. William wrote: ". . . those who are disabled from work by age and invalidity have a well-grounded claim to care from the state."

In Germany, Chancellor Otto von Bismarck, facing the growing threat of Marxism, announced a plan in 1883 to pay any non-working German over 65 a government pension. While this sounds generous, hardly anyone lived to 65 in the 1880s, with most people carried off by injury or disease well before that age. However, his actions led to the establishment of the de facto age of retirement that endures today.

Bismarck was motivated to introduce social insurance in Germany to promote the well-being of workers, keep the German economy operating at maximum efficiency, and avert calls for more radical socialist alternatives. The German system provided contributory retirement benefits and disability benefits as well. Participation was mandatory and contributions were taken from the employee, the employer and the government. Coupled with the workers' compensation program established in 1884 and the "sickness" insurance enacted the year before, this gave the Germans a comprehensive system of income security based on social insurance principles. (They would add unemployment insurance in 1927, making their system complete.)

One persistent myth about the German program is that it adopted age 65 as the standard retirement age because that was Bismarck's age. America also adopted age 65 as retirement benefits because Germany adopted this age when they created their program.[1]

The Origins of the Retirement Age in Social Security in the United States:

When farming dominated the economy of the United States, most men worked as long as their health held out. As they aged, though, they often cut their hours and turned the most physically demanding chores over to sons or hired hands. In 1880, when half of Americans worked on a farm, 78 per cent of American men worked past age 65.

The studies showed that age 65 produced a manageable system that could easily be made self-sustaining with only modest levels of payroll taxation. While the Social Security Act passed in 1935, the official retirement age was 65, but life expectancy for American men was around 58 at the time.

Almost immediately after that, though, that balance changed. The depression ended, and wealth and better medicine meant that Americans started to live longer in the post-war boom. By 1960, life expectancy in America was almost 70 years. Suddenly, more people lived past the age where they had permission to stop working and the money to do it. Finally, they began to retire in sizeable numbers-to stop working, embrace leisure to golf. For a few decades, older Americans lived without working, enough that we've come to expect that we *should* be able to retire, even if that may no longer be financially possible for many. Today, the Social Security Administration estimates 38 million retired people in the United States alone.

According to the Mental Health Foundation, one in five present-day retirees experiences depression. Those living alone because of bereavement or divorce are more at risk. Physical health problems can also make people more vulnerable to mental health issues. Recent studies have indicated that "retirement increases the chances of suffering from clinical depression by around 40 per cent, and of having at least one diagnosed physical illness by 60 per cent". On the other hand, many workers have adopted scaling back on their jobs at around 55 or 60, or even changing careers, but still working for 15-20 more years.

Life after retirement in America:

Retirement age coincides with significant life changes; a retired worker might move to a new location, for example a retirement community, thereby having less frequent contact with their previous social context and adopting a new lifestyle. Often retirees volunteer for charities and other community organizations. Tourism is a standard marker of retirement and, for some becomes a way of life such as for so-called grey nomads. Some retired people even choose to go and live in warmer climates in what is known as retirement migration.

Americans have six lifestyle choices as they age: continuing to work full time, continuing to work part time, retiring from work and becoming engaged in a variety of recreational and leisure activities, retiring from career and later returning to work part time, and retiring from work and later returning to work full time. An important note to make from these lifestyle definitions are that four of the six involve working.[2]

Evolution of retirement in India:

India has complex provident fund and pension schemes targeted at different segments of the labour force. The country's social security system has seven components: the Employee

Provident Fund Organization (EPFO) schemes, civil service schemes, the schemes of public enterprises, superannuation plans of the corporate sector, and voluntary tax-advantaged social assistance schemes, and micro pension schemes. However, formal retirement provisions cover less than 12% of India's 450 million active workforces. Traditionally, access to standard retirement benefits for Indian workers is limited to salaried employees of the central and state governments and those of the larger private and public sector companies. Since most of India's workforce is informal, most Indian workers are not covered by formal retirement programs.

Two principal concerns have driven India's pension reform. The first was a fiscal imperative to truncate the unfunded defined benefit civil service pension scheme covering nearly 25 million central and state government employees. The second was a social imperative to provide a sustainable and scalable pension system to India's informal sector workers. They have not, until the present, enjoying the benefits of a government sponsored retirement income arrangement. Reforming the Pension System on January 1 2004, upon the recommendation of the Project Old Age Social and Income Security Committee, the Government of India embarked on an ambitious pension reform plan. It sought to replace the traditional defined benefit civil service pension scheme with a new defined contribution scheme for government employees by installing the national pension system (NPS) and establishing an interim Pension Fund Regulatory and Development Authority (PFRDA). The government also decided to extend the NPS to India's 400 million informal sector workers, making a unified pension arrangement mandatory for government employees and voluntary for others. Currently, 23 state governments have introduced the NPS scheme for their new employees. Supporting the Implementation of Pension Reforms to help the government implement pension reforms, the Asian Development Bank (ADB) provided its first pension reform-related technical assistance (TA) in 1999. TA covered the overall legal, regulatory, and tax frameworks for the pension and provident funds and supported the strategy for modernizing the EPFO.

The TA helped formulate strategies and measurable action plans and develop and test pension products before rolling them out to formal and informal sectors. The TA also allowed the government and PFRDA to create a database to determine the casual sector workers' demand and ability to pay for voluntary retirement contributions and the nature and the size of the excluded funds. The TA supported in the following areas: Raise awareness regarding workers participation in the NPS; Evaluate the effectiveness of NPS, institutional support mechanisms and the ability of the points of presence to deliver quality services, including sales, promotions, collection, pooling, and transfer of pension savings to the central record-keeping agency and pension fund managers; Assess the effectiveness of service delivery and adequacy of benefits under existing schemes, and develop strategies for effective service delivery; and Study of product development for formulating and field-testing in four selected districts to test market demand and the informal sector workers' ability to pay for such products.[3]

A good 100 million people in India, or a little less than 9% of its population, are over 60 years of age today, and that number will triple by 2050. Meaning, every fifth Indian will be a sexagenarian compared with one in twelve now. And most of them will be financially insecure in their sunset years if a social security net doesn't get built starting from now. And if a large number of the old end up having no pension by 2030, the government will have to bear the heavy fiscal burden of providing minimum sustenance to them. A multi-fold increase in pension coverage to the private sector workforce is, therefore, an imperative.

As per estimates by the United Nations Population Division, this number in India will climb to 180 million (over 12% of the population) by 2030. Further nearly 300 million (over 18%) by

2050. In the next 35 years, people aged 60 or more will multiply 2.6 times, while that those in the working-age bracket of 15-59 will rise by less than half of that. That means there will be only 3.3 workers per older person in 2030 from 4.2 today. The number gets crunched further to 2.4 workers by 2050.

The ageing population is a big worry globally. A Standard & Poor's report (Global Ageing 2013: Rising to the challenge) finds that several countries might need to take unpopular steps to reduce their budgets to accommodate pension support to the ageing population. The analysis suggested that altering demographically driven budget trajectories is equally pressing for both the advanced economies and some emerging market sovereigns. Though the proportion of India's old people is less than those of several developed countries and below the world average, the rise from where we stand today will be steep-hence the need to act fast.

The fiscal cost of ageing (2.2% of GDP at present), the price the government incurs on those beyond the working-age depends on the following factors:

1. Number of pensioners: Available estimates suggest that central (except armed forces pensioners) and state government pensioners will continue to decline. The employment base of the public sector, which will eventually turn into retirees, has been falling in recent years as fresh recruitment has not kept pace with attrition, partly as a deliberate effort to downsize government employment.

2. Nature of pension schemes (employee contributory or non-contributory): The central government has introduced the National Pension System (NPS) scheme for all its employees (except armed forces) recruited after January 1, 2004. NPS requires employees to contribute towards their pension, unlike the previously defined benefit scheme, which is non-contributory, unfunded and wage and inflation-indexed. It will ensure that government pension obligations towards employee pensions will decline after peaking in the 2030s. By 2050, the central

government will only be liable to make pension payments to armed forces' pensioners. At the state level, all states except West Bengal, Tripura and Telangana have adopted NPS.

3. Growth rate of pension per person: Pension per person grows because of dearness allowance granted and one-time rise due to revision in pay scales. While the Pay Commission revisions tend to raise pay scales to accommodate living standards, the dearness allowance is linked to inflation.

4. Six pension schemes for senior citizens offered by the Government of India are i) National Pension System (NPS) scheme ii) Atal Pension Yojana (APY) iii)Pradhana Mantri Vaya Vandana Yojana(PMVVY) iv) Indira Gandhi National Old Age Pension Scheme (IGNOAPS) v) Employee Pension Scheme (EPS) vi) Varishtha Pension Bima Yojana(VPBY).[4]

CHAPTER THREE

Research Studies – Healthy Ageing

Only staying active will make you want to live a hundred years.

- A Japanese proverb

A good life allows maximum independence. Making our life meaningful and purposeful in old age is very important for health and longevity. Health is physical and mental wellbeing. The first thing to be healthy is to be happy. But a single yardstick can not measure happiness. Happiness comes with contentment concerning various issues facing in our day to day life, say money, possessing worldly things including house, furniture, children's education, their placement etc. Mahatma Gandhi said, "Happiness is when what you think, say, and do are in harmony". What does Gandhi's quote mean? "Live as if you were to die tomorrow. Learn as if you were to live forever." - Seize the moment, live without regrets, do what you have to do. Don't postpone things for tomorrow, because tomorrow might not come.[1]

The World Health Organization (WHO) defines ageing as a "process of progressive change in the biological, psychological and social structure of individuals". Yet another definition is "the lifelong process of growing older at the cellular, organ, and whole-body level throughout the life span". Thus, a decline, change or development can be viewed as ageing. A decline in body and mental functions has a negative connotation. A change in body and cognitive functions is neutral in meaning-however, not all aspects of ageing decline with age. Our capacity for joy and ability to love does not diminish, so experience, knowledge, and wisdom can only increase, which has to be supported by good health and memory with time.

One of the reasons for the lack of a singular definition of ageing is that it can be considered in so many different ways, according to social, behavioural, physiological, morphological, cellular and molecular changes and norms. Research has led to several theories being proposed that may explain the ageing process.

Normal ageing:

Many people see ageing as a time of cognitive and physical decline. For the past three decades, the general public and most scientists have accepted this negative age stereotype as the norm. The elderly have been viewed and labelled as 'ill or disabled', 'ugly', 'mentally declining', 'mentally ill', 'isolated', 'poor' and 'depressed'. This negative stereotyping of and discrimination against people because they are old is known as "ageism".

Studies of human ageing in the 1960s to 1980s focused on average "normal" age-related functional losses with ageing in organs and systems of the body. While it is true that bodily functions degrade as we get old, we have all seen people who look younger and are more capable than their peers. This has even been scientifically documented. The traditional ageing research neglected this, despite evidence that there are substantial functional differences in older persons within the same age groups. Differences in functionality within age groups were simply attributed to genetic endowment. Although genetic factors contribute to the way we age and is a field of research on its own, our genes still only account for a minor part of how gracefully we age. Twin studies that examined the influence of genes on ageing have shown that heritability explains about 20-30% of differences in lifespan and 22% of differences in functioning. Both longevity and functioning appear less heritable than cognitive ability. Thus, most of the differences between how gracefully we age stem from non-heritable influences of peoples environment and lifestyle, which are not part of the ageing process.

Healthy ageing:

Such a grouping of ageing processes de-emphasizes the view that ageing is exclusively characterized by declines in functional competence and health and re-focuses on the substantial heterogeneity among old persons. It also underscores the existence of positive outcomes (i.e. without disability, disease, or significant physiological decline). It highlights the possible avoidance of many, if not all, illnesses and disabilities usually associated with old age.

According to the classic definition, successful ageing can be characterized as involving three components: a) Freedom of disease and disability, b) High physical and cognitive functioning c) Social and productive engagement or occupation.

Later refinements to the definition have added psychosocial aspects, such as self-acceptance, positive relations with others, autonomy, purpose in life, food habits and food quality, exercises, mental stress and personal growth. It has also been suggested that successful ageing is a developmental process that can be achieved at any stage in the life span. Regardless of what criteria and what terms we use, we all want to have the capacity to thrive and prosper for as long as we live.

Healthy life expectancy and longevity:

The average lifespan of humans has increased over the past century, mainly as a result of significant improvements in sanitary conditions, public health reforms and improved personal hygiene, advances in medical knowledge and practices, and living standards. At birth, the average life expectancy is now approximately 75 years in males and 80 years in females in the USA (World Health Organization 2003). It can be compared to 48 years at the beginning of the twentieth century.

In the United States, the population aged 65 and older was 4 per cent of the total population in 1900; in 1950, this number had increased to 8.1 per cent, and in 2000 it grew to 12.4 per cent of the total population. The older population in the U.S. grew from 3 million in 1900 to 39 million in 2008, accounting for 13 per cent of the total population.

One of the World Health Organization studies classifies elderly adults between 65 and 74 as youngest-old, those 75-84 as middle old and those over 85 as oldest-old. The oldest-old population that age grew from just over 100,000 in 1900 to 5.7 million in 2008. The number of older people will increase dramatically during the 2010–2030 period. The older population in 2030 is projected to be twice as large as their counterparts in 2000, growing from 35 million to 72 million and representing nearly 20 per cent of the total U.S. population. The oldest-old population is projected to multiply after 2030. The U.S. Census Bureau projects that the population age 85 and over could grow from 5.7 million in 2008 to 19 million by 2050. Some researchers predict that death rates at older generations will decline more rapidly than is reflected in the U.S. Census Bureau's projections, which could lead to even faster growth of this population.

India is ranked the second in the world in terms of its population, with 1.388 b people in 2021. This is around 17.7 per cent of the world's population. India is expected to be the world's most populous country by 2025, outstripping China, according to a UN report, "World population prospects", published in 2012. In 2011 more than 60 per cent of India's population was 15-59 years old. This is a demographic dividend of which the country is proud. However, at the same time, the percentage of its population above 60 years is increasing every year due to improved longevity, driven by an enhanced focus on health care, rising income levels and a better standard of living in the country. By 2030, 12 per cent of India's population will be in the age bracket of 60+ years, which translates into 180 million people- a vast population that is higher than that of many developed countries. The growth rate of the elderly population in India is higher than its general population. This makes the trend of gradual ageing of its population similar to what is observed in other countries. According to the Population Census2011, there are nearly 104 million older people (aged 60 years or above) in India. A report released by the United Nations Population Fund and HelpAge India says that the number of elderly people is expected to grow to 173 million in another eight years and 20 % of the total population by 2050.

Two critical areas in which personal ageing and capabilities can be strengthened:

First - Maintaining independence and engagement alone can account for differences of 10 years of healthy life expectancy. Second- Limiting modifiable risk factors concerning chronic disease is essential. Cardiovascular diseases (CVDs) are the world's leading causes of death and disability, and modifiable risk factors account for most CVD-related deaths. The recent WHO global health risks report lists modifiable risk factors for improving health for life: unsafe use of alcohol and tobacco, high blood pressure, high body mass index (BMI), low intake of fruits and vegetables, and physical inactivity. Together these account for 60% of all global cardiovascular deaths.

The World Health Organization recognized that quality of life in old age is as important as increased longevity and introduced the concept of healthy life expectancy (also called HALE), defined as the number of years an individual is expected to live without any major debilitating diseases. The healthy life expectancy is about 67 years for males and 71 years for females (World Health Organization 2000).

The maximum observed lifespan represents the longest-lived member(s) of the population. In humans, the oldest individual ever recorded was a woman who died in 1997 in France at 122 years. The oldest recorded man died in 1998 at the age of 115. By contrast, the average lifespan (or life expectancy at birth) refers to how long people live on average in a given population. The theoretical maximum lifespan, or potential maximum lifespan, is the academic highest attainable age. Today, we don't know what age this is, but it has been speculated to be around 125 years. Psychological age is how old one feels, acts, and behaves, and is thus not necessarily equal to chronological age, which is an age since birth. Therefore, a person can have a psychological age that exceeds their chronological age if they mature or feel older than they are. Psychological age incorporates attitudes, emotions and cognitive abilities.

United Nations (UN) document says happiness is a mental or emotional state of wellbeing characterized by positive or pleasant emotions ranging from contentment to intense joy. The General Assembly of the United Nations, in its resolution 66/281 of 12 July 2012, proclaimed 20 March the International Day of Happiness, recognizing the relevance of happiness and wellbeing as universal goals and aspirations in the lives of human beings around the world and the importance of their recognition in public policy objectives. It also recognized the need for a more inclusive, equitable, and balanced approach to economic growth that promotes sustainable development, poverty eradication, happiness, and all peoples' wellbeing.

Happiness and health do not come from medicine but peace of mind, heart, and soul. One of the greatest mysteries of human life is ageing or how to prevent the natural ageing process. The medical fraternity focuses on the repair of health but not sustenance of spirit for living. It is observed that one lives longer, only when one stops trying to live longer.

Past research, done in 2013 by the department of psychology, Boise State University, USA, suggests that senior citizens' physical and mental health and quality of life improved when they volunteered to work. Another 2014 study by Baycrest Health Sciences in Canada and published online in 'Psychological Bulletin' found that older adults who stayed active by volunteering improved overall health.

Depressive symptoms negate the benefits of exercise:
Research studies have shown that sound mental health is the key to a happier and longer life. A research paper by P L Lee, published in the International Journal of Aging and Human Development in 2013 found that the popularly known research

evidence that exercise promotes longevity is untrue. If we have symptoms of depression but still exercise, exercise's longevity inspiring effects are nullified. In other words, we could exercise regularly in the sunset years of our life, but if we do not feel mentally strong, we will not enjoy the benefits of a longer life. Possessing mental and physical health should be everyone's priority.[2]

Helping others can add years to our life:

A 20- year-long study of survival data for more than 500 people aged 70-103 years recently published in the Journal of Evolution and Human Behavior found that people who occasionally watched and cared for others lived longer than people who did not. The subjects in the study were grandparents who were not primary caregivers for their grandchildren but still took care of them on an occasional basis. The researchers also looked at people without children who took care of other people. The researchers found that grandparents who watched their grandchildren, and older adults who helped their adult children, were more likely to be alive ten years after their first interview at the start of the study. Among the people who did not provide this type of care, half of the group died five years after the beginning of the study.

Several studies have looked at the link between grandparents and more extended living. Some studies have shown that caregiving can improve a grandparent's cognitive functioning and risk for depression. But the new study's authors have shown that caregiving may provide a health benefit for people even outside of family ties. About half lived for seven years after the initial interview among older adults who provided care for someone in their social network—the people who didn't only live an average of four years later. The researchers believe positive emotions experienced from helping others may combat the negative effects of emotions like stress. More research will be needed to understand the complete mechanisms that underline the health benefits of helping others.[3]

Healthy older adults can generate new brain cells as younger people:

Researchers have found for the first time that healthy older adults can generate just as many new brain cells as younger people. There has been controversy over whether adult humans grow new neurons, and some research has previously suggested that the adult brain was hard-wired and that adults did not grow new neurons. The new study, published in the journal Cell Stem Cell, counters that notion. The findings suggest that many senior citizens remain more cognitively and emotionally intact than commonly believed, said Maura Boldrini, an associate professor at Columbia University in the US. "We found that older people have similar ability to make thousands of hippocampus new neurons from progenitor cells as younger people do," Boldrini said. "We also found equivalent volumes of the hippocampus (a brain structure used for emotion and cognition) across ages. Researchers, including those from New York State Psychiatric Institute, found that even the oldest brains they studied produced new brain cells."[4]

Loneliness is harmful to health:

While loneliness is increasingly recognized as a social issue, what's less well recognized is the role loneliness plays as a critical determinant of health. According to former Surgeon General Vivek Murthy, Loneliness can be deadly, among others, who has stressed the significant health threat. Loneliness has been estimated to shorten a person's life by 15 years, equivalent in impact to being obese or smoking 15 cigarettes per day. A recent study revealed a surprising association between loneliness and cancer mortality risk, pointing to the role loneliness plays in cancer's course, including responsiveness to treatments.

Biologists have shown that feelings of loneliness trigger the release of stress hormones associated with higher blood pressure, decreased resistance to infection, and increased risk of cardiovascular disease and cancer. There's even evidence that this perceived sense of social isolation accelerates cognitive and functional decline and can serve as a preclinical sign for Alzheimer's disease.

The number of people who perceive themselves to be alone, isolated, or distant from others has reached epidemic levels in the United States and other parts of the world. Indeed, almost two decades ago, the book Bowling Alone pointed to the increasing isolation of Americans and our consequent loss of "social capital." In Japan, for example, an estimated half-million (known as hikikomori) shut themselves away for months on end. In the United Kingdom, four in 10 citizens report feelings of chronic, profound loneliness, prompting a new cabinet-level position (the Minister for Loneliness) to combat the problem.

It has long been recognized that social support—through the availability of nutritious food, safe housing and job opportunities- positively influences mental and physical health. Studies have repeatedly shown that those with fewer social connections have the highest mortality rates, highlighting that social isolation can threaten health by lacking access to clinical care, social services or needed support.

So what can be done to combat widespread loneliness and social instability? The good news is that there are models of success already in place in the U.S. and worldwide. Programs such as Meals on Wheels and help-lines that arrange phone calls between volunteers and the lonely—whether they be older adults or teens in crisis-offer direct social support to those feeling profoundly isolated. Intergenerational initiatives, like the dementia-friendly villages in the Netherlands, the Intergenerational Learning Center in Seattle, and global home-sharing programs offer unique opportunities for the elderly to make meaningful connections with children and young adults.[5]

Doing household chores is as good as going to the gym:

A study tracking 13000 people in 17 countries, both rich and poor, found that whether going to the gym, walking to work, or tackling household chores like laundry or gardening, being physically active extends life and reduces illness. Researchers said that one in 12 global deaths over five years could be prevented through 30 minutes of physical activity, including house-cleaning or walking to work- five days a week. "Being highly active (750 minutes a week) is associated with an even greater reduction." According to a study published in "The Lancer" medical journal.

The study confirms that physical activity is associated with a lower risk of mortality and cardiovascular disease on a global scale. The authors said this was irrespective of which country the study participants came from, the type of activity or whether it was undertaken for leisure or as part of daily transport or housework.

World Health Organization (WHO) recommends at least 150 minutes of "moderate-intensity" or 75 minutes of "vigorous-intensity" aerobic physical activity per week. According to the study authors, almost a quarter of the world population does not meet this requirement. The new study showed that "walking for as little as 30 minutes most days of the week has substantial benefit", said the lead author Scott Lear of the Simon Fraser University in Canada.

The study included participants aged 35 to 70 from urban and rural areas in rich and developing nations. They were followed over nearly seven years. The researchers noted how many suffered heart attacks, stroke or heart failure, among other diseases and compared these figures to the individual's physical activity levels. "Of the 106,970 people who met the activity guidelines, 3.8 % developed cardiovascular diseases, compared to 5.1% of people who did not," said authors.[6]

Compression of Morbidity theory:

Compression of morbidity refers to reducing the length of time a person spends sick or disabled to maximize a healthy lifespan. The term was first coined by Dr. James Fries, professor of medicine at Stanford University, in 1980. Dr. Fries theorized that most illnesses are chronic and occur near the end of life. If the onset of these chronic illnesses could be delayed, the healthy time saved could lessen the burden of disease over a person's lifetime. Compression of morbidity has become one of the goals of healthy ageing and longevity: living disease-free and illness-free for as long as possible.

The compression of morbidity is like this: if a person's life expectancy is 80 years, but they develop diabetes and congestive heart failure at age 60, that person will spend some 20 years with serious chronic conditions that likely will impact their ability to live independently and enjoy life. Suppose the person adopts a healthier lifestyle and delays diabetes and congestive heart failure until age 70. In that case, that person will have compressed the "sick" time into a much shorter period.

It is possible that adopting a healthier lifestyle earlier could increase the person's life expectancy, too. Still, medical research has shown it may not increase lifespan more than a few years. Therefore, the main idea is to shrink the bad months and years between illness/disability and death.

A study was done at Stanford that examined the risk factors and morbidity/disability in 418 adults over 12 years. The study concluded age-related morbidity could be reduced and postponed with healthier lifestyles. For individuals, Dr. Fries and his colleagues recommend a strategy that involves staying active, never smoking, and never becoming obese (losing weight if you are overweight or obese). That is the health advice we will probably find familiar.

"Fries hypothesis" holds that if the age at the onset of the first chronic infirmity (disease) can be postponed more rapidly than the age of death, then the lifetime illness burden may be compressed into a shorter period nearer to the age of death. Evidence supporting this hypothesis thus must take two forms: first, it is possible to delay the onset of infirmity substantially; second, the accompanying increases in longevity will be comparatively modest. The idea behind compression of morbidity is to squeeze or compress the time horizon between the onset of chronic illness or disability and when a person dies.

James Fries is the author of more than 300 articles, numerous book chapters, and 11 books, including *Take Care of Yourself* and *Living Well.* According to him, by minimizing the number of years people suffer from chronic illness, we enable older people to live more successful, productive lives that benefit them and society. When we consider healthcare reform and new approaches to structuring health care systems, we must recognize that by avoiding long-term periods of morbidity, we reduce healthcare costs and improve patients' lives at the same time.

Since Fries' seminal article on his hypothesis was published in *The New England Journal of Medicine*, compression of morbidity has been intensely discussed and argued for nearly three decades. Today, with data strongly confirming the hypothesis, compression of morbidity has become widely recognized as the dominant paradigm for healthy ageing at both individual and policy levels. It is thought to have laid the foundation for successful health promotion and programs.

Fries a Philosopher-Cum-Physician:

Although Fries is one of America's most well-known and respected rheumatologists and an expert on long-term outcomes, he did not always want to be a physician. Fries studied philosophy as an undergraduate at Stanford. He describes himself as a young man interested in the "great thoughts" on which classical philosophy is based: *Why are we here? How do we define the human condition?* He surprised himself when he began to find the answers to these questions in the study of medicine.

In his studies, he began to believe that the possibility of understanding life through forces of reason and without data had been exhausted. Instead, he began to think that a greater understanding of life and death would come from the data of biological sciences and, in particular, medicine.

After a brief period as a philosophy instructor at Stanford, Fries headed to Johns Hopkins School of Medicine. He graduated with a degree in internal medicine and completed a fellowship in rheumatology. Fries explained, "As a field of study and practice, rheumatology was an excellent blend of things I wanted and was interested in. I had the opportunity to watch life course events in patients with rheumatologic disease and the diseases were chronic and intellectually exciting to me. They also involved the art of dealing with the person and the science of projecting long-term outcomes. It was here that I really developed an interest in moving medicine and healthcare in general from short-term outcomes to long-term outcomes."

The Genesis of a New Model:

Fries joined the Stanford faculty in 1970. He formulated the compression of morbidity hypothesis during his first sabbatical from 1978 to 1979 at the Center for Advanced Studies and Behavior Sciences, an independent research institution in Stanford, California. Ageing was the centre's theme that academic year and improving senior capabilities from several perspectives were the focus of the fellows' discussion.

We entered the twentieth century in an era of acute infectious diseases, with tuberculosis the number one killer of our population and smallpox, diphtheria, tetanus, and other contagious illnesses comprising 80% of all deaths in 1900. With these diseases nearly eradicated by the 1970s, mortality from these diseases has been reduced by nearly 99%, ushering in an era where the major burdens of illness in the United States are chronic diseases—heart disease, stroke, cancer, and diabetes.

As life expectancy steadily rose and patterns of disease experienced a profound shift, the prevailing mythology at the time suggested an unfortunate scenario for future health. As medical progress increasingly prolonged life, those extra months and years would be spent in ill health. This theory, termed "the failure of success," assumed that although advances in medicine and public health could prolong life, they could not delay the onset of chronic, degenerative diseases.

Paradigm Shift:

The compression of morbidity hypothesis presented a new lens through which to examine ageing- that viewed prevention, lifestyle changes, and health improvements as the keys to delaying the onset of morbidity. Fries said, "In contrast to what many demographers and health policy workers of the time believed, the compression of morbidity hypothesis represented a positive concept, with the idea of a long life with a relatively short period of terminal decline."

James Fries has made a more significant contribution than anyone else in the understanding that there is a way to be free of health problems until the very end of life and how important this is in health care costs and quality of life each of us can enjoy.

Proof of Concept:

Over the past 20 years, the compression of morbidity hypothesis has generated a tremendous amount of research, including rigorous, longitudinal studies through the Arthritis, Rheumatism and Aging Medical Information System (ARAMIS), a databank established by Fries and funded by the National Institutes of Health as the National Arthritis Data Resource. ARAMIS includes two large longitudinal studies of ageing directed at quantification of the compression of morbidity hypothesis to demonstrate the effect of health promotion and prevention in delaying the onset of morbidity.

The first of the studies followed 1700 University of Pennsylvania alumni for 20 years to determine whether people with lower modifiable health risks have a more or less cumulative disability. After adjusting for possible confounding variables, they found that the cumulative lifetime disability was four times greater in those who smoked, were obese, and did not exercise than in those who did not smoke, lean, and exercise. The onset of measurable disability was postponed by nearly 8 years in the lowest-risk third of the study participants compared with the highest-risk third.

Further support for the compression of morbidity hypothesis came from a second 22-year longitudinal study. Participants were

537 members of a runners' club and 423 community control participants who were 59 years old on average. They found that the runners developed disability at a rate of only one fourth that of the control participants and were able to postpone disability by more than 12 years over the more sedentary control participants.

The hypothesis developed by Fries, a gifted physician dedicated to quality care, is expected to hold in the years ahead, as long as society continues to emphasize healthy lifestyles, further improvements in preventive medicine, and a better living environment for the elderly. "We cannot compress morbidity indefinitely, but the paradigm of a long, healthy life with a relatively rapid terminal decline is most certainly an attainable ideal at both a population level and individual level," said Fries.

Health policies must be directed at modifying those health risks that precede and cause morbidity if compression of morbidity is applied to a population. At an individual level, there are three key issues Americans need to pay attention to when it comes to health and postponing morbidity-smoking, obesity, and exercise.

Fries, a role model -lives by his word:

Although James Fries, the father of two children (one deceased) and five grandchildren, maintains that there is no one way to compress morbidity, he suggests everything in moderation, except physical activity, which he stresses as the key to delaying the onset of morbidity. Fries heeds his advice, having run at least 500 miles each year since 1970. He has also completed the Boston Marathon and is a high-altitude climber who has reached the peak of the tallest summit on six of the seven continents.

Whatever James undertakes will be done efficiently, effectively and quickly. James takes on challenges few others will take, such as climbing Mt. Everest, [participating in] adventure travelling, or horseback riding with his wife, Sarah, in [Botswana's] Okavango Delta.

Together, Fries and Sarah have led an active life, skiing and adventure, travelling worldwide, from the North Pole to Southeast Asia. Today, Fries is also a caregiver for Sarah, a long-term melanoma (a type of skin cancer) survivor and living with a disability. Fries said, "I have a surprising amount of satisfaction in helping to care for Sarah, and together we have done many things, especially after her illness, that people said we would not, that people believed were not possible."

In February, Fries and Sarah celebrated the 50th anniversary of their first kiss and have been married nearly as long. "Do I have any words of wisdom? Remember that there is no one magic pathway to living a happy life of longevity and vitality. But there are endless possibilities and we can all have a substantial effect upon our future health," said Fries.[7]

Why should companies recruit people over 50 for senior and responsible positions?

Because they are more productive than those below50! A massive study in America found that most of the productive age in man's life is 60-70. From 70-80 is the second most productive age. The third most productive age is 50-60. The average of a Nobel Prize winner is 62. The average of a CEO in a Fortune 500 company is 63. The average age of Pope's age is 76. This tells us somehow; God has designed that the best years of your life are 60-80! It is when you do your best work. A study published in NEJM found that at 60, you reach your peak of political and continues up to 80! So, if you are between 60-70 or 70-80, you have the best and second-best years of life with you.[8]

70-79 years old is a dangerous period:

Israeli scholars have found that there are around two health problems per month for elderly people between the ages of 70 and 79. Surprisingly, the health status of the elderly aged 80-89 is as stable as the 60-69 age groups. 70-79 years old is a dangerous period. During this period, various organs decline rapidly. It is a frequent period of various geriatric diseases, and it is often prone to Hyperlipidemia (blood has too many lipids or fats), arteriosclerosis, hypertension and diabetes. After entering the age of 80, these diseases will decline, and the mental and physical health may return to the level of 60-69 years old. Thus, the age of 70-79 years old is called the 'dangerous age group". As people grow older many people want to have a good healthy life. They realize that 'Health is Wealth'. Hence, the 10 -year health care of 70-79 years old is crucial.[9]

CHAPTER FOUR

Lifelong Learning for Longevity

What Is Lifelong Learning?

Humans learn over their entire lifespan. Learning, in general, can occur in various contexts, which are commonly divided into formal, non-formal and informal settings. At the same time, formal learning occurs within a traditional hierarchical and chronological education system and typically finishes with a degree or credential. Non-formal learning consists of organised and systematic educational activities presented to selected population groups, such as older adults, who do not lead towards a degree or credential. Informal learning takes place outside of these contexts and can be understood as a non-intentional and often unconscious form of learning, like learning from experience. The majority of organised education for older adults occurs in the context of non-formal learning.

Why Is Lifelong Learning Important?

Many developed countries globally, including the United States, experience ageing of their populations, which results in a reversal of the population's age structure. Important factors for this global population growth and ageing are decreasing fertility, declining mortality rate, and an increased life expectancy due to improvements in public health and health care. While the number of adults in retirement age increases, the number of individuals in working-age decreases (demographic change). After retirement has developed into an independent and expanded life stage, the individual can expect to spend more than twenty years in retirement. These developments consequently lead to how the workforce and current retirement systems can be maintained in the future and how retirement time can be filled with meaning. As a strategy, society and educational politics need to increasingly acknowledge and utilise the skills and knowledge of the elderly as an important resource as well as provide possibilities for ongoing participation in organised education and professional development over the life span.

Switzerland has legislation following individuals who continue to work up to five years beyond the statutory retirement age to increase their state pension at the time of withdrawal. The Norwegian government has pursued a national lifelong learning initiative known as Competence Reform. Employees who have worked at least three years for the same employer during the last two years have the right to full or part-time study leave for up to three years. This initiative aims to provide the country with a highly-skilled, flexible workforce. Competence Reform will also aid in the knowledge transfer of new technologies and help older workers remain competitive in the workforce. The Japanese government offers companies incentives to encourage older workers to stay in the workforce, including subsidies whose total workforce has more than 10% older workers and employers who have eliminated mandatory retirement.

What Makes Older Adults as Learners Special?

Characteristic for learning in older adulthood is a high level of autonomy and self-directedness. While learning at a younger age often occurs in mandatory and specific institutional settings, (older) adult learning is much more voluntary and driven by intrinsic motivation rather than external factors. In addition, the individual biography and life experiences gain relevance for learning with increasing age. Since the individual tends only to know what appears to be relevant and integral, learning at an older age can therefore be understood as a highly individualised and self-structured process, for which the learner is self-responsible. However, older adults learn differently from younger individuals as the brain and memory functions are subject to ageing processes. A decreasing functionality of short-term memory affects learning abilities in old age. Learning processes become more prone to interference, and recently learned items may be harder to recall.[1]

Learning is something we do throughout our entire lives. We don't simply stop learning once we finish school – we learn new things every day. The learning we do in adulthood isn't always done in a classroom, but it still counts! Think about all the new things we learn in a day, whether it's at work, learning a new skill in the kitchen, or reading about something online. Learning is an essential part of life and is something we should all seek to continue as we get older.

Learning new things becomes especially important in the senior years. It's a great way to keep the mind and body active and play a big part in keeping seniors happy and healthy. Whether in a more formal classroom setting or just learning something new from a friend, it's good to encourage our loved ones to seek knowledge. Let's take a look at why learning is as important as we age. It's essential to keep the brain active as we get older. Learning new skills or about new subjects is a great way to keep the mind sharp. Continued learning can improve memory by maintaining brain cells and ensuring those cells properly communicate with each other. Think of your mind as a muscle; it needs to be exercised regularly to keep it strong.

Learning something new is a great way to boost self-esteem. When you know a new skill, you feel stronger, more confident, and proud of yourself. New skills can give you a stronger sense of independence, which will keep you happy and healthy. One study suggests that the belief that you are smart and have a strong mind can help prevent memory loss. In the study, older people did worse on memory-related tasks after being exposed to negative stereotypes about seniors and forgetfulness. They performed better on those same tasks when they were told that it's possible to preserve your memory well into your later years.

When we decide to attend a class or lecture, we will be surrounded by people who share common interests. For example, if we choose to take a course on speaking a new language, we know everyone is interested in learning the same thing. It is a built-in ice breaker - chat with everyone about why they're excited to learn this new skill.

It allows us to make new friends outside of the classroom too. Organise a study group to keep in touch with our fellow students, or get together to talk about what we have learned. We will likely open the door to some amazing new friends who will keep us busy and entertained.

Once we retire, we have the gift of free time. It's the perfect opportunity to take that course we always wanted to take or pick up that hobby we always wanted to try out. The satisfaction of finally mastering that skill or digging into a subject we have always been curious about will give us a massive boost of self-confidence, and we will feel great about making good use of our free time.[2]

How Physical Activity Helps the Brain

Here we can adhere to the old adage "Use it or lose it." Walking, yoga, swimming—we're all familiar with the general health benefits of exercise. But how aware are we with the idea that physical exercise does as much for the brain as it does the body? As a general rule, as we get older, the hippocampus (the area of the brain involved in learning and memory) shrinks one to two per cent annually in people without dementia. However, studies have found that this trend can be stopped and, in many cases, even reversed. Physical activity stimulates specific brain areas and even increases the birth of new nerve cells in the hippocampus. It defies outright the age-old belief that our brains are static and that once we lose a brain cell, it's gone for good. A study conducted at the University of Illinois clearly showed how modest but regular aerobic exercise can improve overall cognitive health. Older adults who participated in the study took

40-minute walks three days per week for one year. In that year alone, the participants saw a two-per cent increase in the size of their hippocampus.[3]

The World Health Organization (WHO) endorsed the Active Ageing Framework in 2002. It has influenced ageing policies and practices worldwide and drawn public attention to the new opportunities and challenges that global ageing brings to individuals and societies. The active ageing framework advocates optimising opportunities for 'health', 'participation' and 'security' – three critical determinants of the quality of retired life. It also supports recognising physical health, mental health and social connections as equally important elements (WHO 2002). Active ageing discourse results from growing governmental concerns about financing health care and social services for ageing populations. At the same time, it mirrors and potentially promotes a positive shift in social attitudes towards old age: viewing later life not as a period of deficits, but as either a time of competency and knowledge or a period of opportunity and wellbeing, with retention or development of the psychological and cognitive resources to cope with life's challenges. [4]

Research studies on lifelong learning:

Research suggests that continuous learning provides numerous benefits for the older individual concerning cognitive functioning, health and wellbeing, civic participation, and self-confidence.

1) A study conducted in 1999 for the American Association of Retired Persons (AARP) by Roper Starch Worldwide, Inc indicated that more than 90% of surveyed adults aged 50 and older planned to continue learning as they age. When asked why respondents indicated they wanted to keep up with what's going on in the world and continue their personal and spiritual growth and experience the fun of learning something new. Lifelong learning is really about the ways to keep the mind, body, and spirit stimulated, challenged, and fully engaged after retirement. There are good reasons to do so. Research during the 1990s, a decade of pioneering brain research, proved that a stimulated

mind promotes a healthy brain. Studies show that keeping brains stimulated helps elders retain mental alertness as they age. The brain's physical anatomy responds to enriching mental activities. Scientists have discovered that even an ageing brain can grow new connections and pathways when challenged and stimulated.

2) In the words of Paul Nussbaum, PhD, director of the Aging Research and Education Center in Pittsburgh, "Every time your heart beats, 25% of that blood goes right to the brain. But while exercise is critical, it may be education that is more important. In the 21st century, education and information may become for the brain what exercise is for the heart." Just like the human heart, our brains need to be nurtured. So think of lifelong learning as a health club for ageing brains.

Along with keeping the brain alert and stimulated as we age, we are also aware of the importance of keeping the body active. Lifelong learning can help in this area as well. Different programs offer opportunities to incorporate activity into daily living. For instance, spirituality, meditation, group singing, participation in prayers, yoga, the exercise of all types, the creative arts, walking clubs, senior citizens clubs and enjoying nature outdoors are only a few of the many opportunities available. Many older adults participate in lifelong learning programs for the social aspects and the learning experience. Outdoor programs, field trips, luncheons, parties, and travel far and near provide opportunities to make new friends engage in stimulating discussions and share life's ups and downs with like-minded people. Making lifelong learning part of the later years fosters a sense of personal empowerment and increased self-esteem. It ensures continued growth and intellectual stimulation, leading to a more fulfilling, enjoyable, and enriched lifestyle. Equally important is the enhanced quality of life. It helps develop natural abilities, immerses in the wonders of life, stimulates natural curiosity about the world, increases wisdom, enables individuals to use their experiences to make the world a better place, and helps them face inevitable societal changes. [5]

3) Healthier brains: Learning something new, such as a new skill or hobby, can help boost our memory. Neuroscientists at the University of Texas at Dallas conducted a study that found that seniors who took on a new mentally challenging hobby saw a lasting increase in their memory skills. These researchers believe that taking on a new challenging activity—like learning to quilt, play an instrument, or operate a computer, for example—strengthens numerous networks within the brain.

4) A research study conducted by neurologists at Case Western Reserve University in Cleveland, US found that engaging in a lifelong pursuit of mentally challenging activities may help prevent Alzheimer's disease. The study found that seniors who frequently read, played mentally tough games like chess, or engaged in other intellectually stimulating activities are 2.5 times less likely to have Alzheimer's, impacting approximately 4 million Americans.

5) Another study of Massachusetts General Hospital and Harvard Medical School also had similar findings. The researchers found, using participant's interviews and brain scans, that seniors who reported higher levels of intellectual stimulation throughout their lifetimes had a significant delay in the onset of memory problems or other Alzheimer's-type symptoms. The ability to delay or even prevent the potentially debilitating symptoms of Alzheimer's offers substantial advantages to the quality of life of senior citizens.

6) Pursuing lifelong learning activities has benefits that go beyond boosting your brainpower. Cognitive neuropsychologists at the University of Sussex in England did a study that found that reading for even just six minutes lowered study participants' stress levels, slowing their heart rates and easing tension in their muscles. And lower stress has wide ranging benefits for seniors' cardiovascular health, decreasing blood pressure and reducing the risk of a stroke or heart attack, boosting immunity, and lowering levels of depression.

7) Researchers at Harvard and Princeton had even more impressive findings in their research on the connection between lifelong learning and health. The study authors found that one more year of education increased life expectancy by 0.18 years. They discovered that the more educated a person, the lower their rates of anxiety and depression as well as the most common acute and chronic diseases (heart disease, stroke, hypertension, high cholesterol, emphysema, diabetes, asthma, ulcer), and they were far less likely to report that they were in overall poor health.[6]

8) The Rush Memory and Aging Project, conducted in 2012 in Chicago with more than 1,200 elders participating, showed that increased cognitive activity in older adults slowed their decline in cognitive function and decreased their risk of mild cognitive impairment. The study showed that cognitively active seniors, whose average age was 80, were 2.6 times less likely to develop Alzheimer's disease and dementia than seniors with less cognitive activity.

My Endeavour for Learning:

Earning a PhD at 61 - I have had a passion for overseas assignments in some United Nations or some Non-Government organisations in agriculture and rural development since my joining bank service. In this direction, I used to see advertisements in journals like The Economist and other related websites. In one such attempt, one of my colleagues in NABARD, Dr. K.S.Viswanatham went to Eritrea, a small African nation, first as a water management expert, next as Associate Dean and Professor of water resources engineering in the College of Agriculture at Asmara. Later on, he also worked for UNDP in the Middle East as a water resource management expert. He was receiving remuneration in USD, and substantial tax-free savings could be repatriated to India. So he suggested applying for teaching posts of Professor and Associate Professor Positions. While facing the interview in January 2005 at Pune, the recruiters told me that they could take me only for Associate Professor Post since I do not have a PhD and as donors insist that a professor should have doctoral qualification. But I was not ready to accept the offer though there was not much difference in remuneration. At the same time, suddenly, I thought that I should continue my studies for a PhD. I was 58, then two years left for retirement. Some people commented why I should pursue PhD at fag end of my retirement with neither increment nor promotion by adding another qualification.

When I rejected the offer of Associate Professor Post, then and there itself, I decided to study for a PhD. When Dr. Viswanatham came to know about my decision, he extended his helping hand. Since I was in service, I was not able to attend regular PhD classes. Hence I thought of some distance education universities in Maharashtra as I was in Pune. Dr. Viswanatham telephoned his friends and found out that Yeshwantrao Chavan Maharashtra Open University (YCMOU), Nashik offers a 3- year PhD course in Agricultural Development. I had planned to go to the United States to visit my daughter in April for three months. So I visited Nashik to know my eligibility and admission procedures. As per age and qualification, I was eligible, but the admission was on a first-come, first-serve basis, and the application form was to be issued on June 1, and the last submission date was June 5. I cut short my US visit so that I could submit my application on time. I was in Nashik the previous day itself to enable me to stand in the queue at 1 AM on June 1. On the same day, I submitted my duly filled application.

As I was eligible, I got admission to the 3- year course, which consisted of 1- year course work and 2 -year research work. But I had to attend regular classes for three days in the YCMOU campus at Nashik once in 2 months on weekends from Friday to Sunday. I studied very hard by answering the model question papers and writing the answers to keep the speed in the final exam. The exam was conducted under very strict invigilators. One of the very senior students asked to leave the examination hall. The invigilator shouted at the student, "You are a professor. Is it not? Why are you copying? Get out. You are debarred from this examination". Thank God! I took the studies very seriously and passed with first class. As a part of this course, we had to submit four assignments on different topics, out of which two cases had to be published in recognised journals. I chose one research topic titled "BAIF's Orchard (*Wadi*) Development Programme in relation to socio-economic transformation of tribal areas in Maharashtra". BAIF is a Non-Government Organization based in Pune which adopted a holistic approach for the poor tribal community by following principles: Awareness building, community mobilisation, grass-root level institution building for sustainability, participatory planning, mentoring, human approach to development, transparency in dealing with farmers, ownership of community assets by the community, employing local field guides, local health workers and barefoot accountants, committed supervisory staff at every level. The thesis was submitted within three years, and I got PhD at 61 after my retirement.

Later the thesis was also published as a book because the findings were so impressive and relevant that people wanted to replicate this model in other states. By adding a PhD, I could serve in very senior positions as a full-time employee for ten years after retirement and as a freelance consultant even today. You will find details here in the last chapter. Incidentally, I would like to mention that I had three very respectable professors who taught my PhD course and bear the name Surya (sun) viz. Dr. Somnath Suryawanshi, Dr.Surya Gunjal and Dr.Suryabhan Sananse. Among them, Dr. Somnath Suryawanshi was my PhD guide, senior by age, experience, and mentored me to become a professor later. These professors also treated me as a good friend. It encouraged me to become an academic student and come up with a better outcome.

Six-month course on Lay-Counselling at 72:

Lifelong learning is the best form of retention of cognitive power. Activities are necessary to maintain a life quality. No matter one's age, people who remain active in all respects-physically, mentally, and socially adjust better for the ageing process. Acceptance of changes seems to link to wellbeing. They develop the capacity to accept life's vagaries, and they are resilient in the face of adversity. I joined a Lay Counselling course offered by Prasanna Counselling Centre, Bangalore, to keep my cognitive power intact. Lay Counsellor brings empathy, a listening ear and natural helping abilities to help seekers. The main job of the Counsellor is to bridge the gap between the patient and the doctor. Research studies on ageing reveal that keeping fit both body and mind are prerequisites for maintaining good health. By learning new things, one can keep the cognitive power of the brain very sharp.

The spirit behind the Prasanna Counselling Centre is octogenarian M C Pankaja, co-founder of Bangalore's oldest counselling centre. She has devoted her life to making psychological help accessible to thousands of people free of charge. At the age of 87, with a spinal cord that has degenerated to cause a hunch of the back, M C Pankaja still walks into her office every day to not miss a day of work of 3 hours. She reaches Prasanna Counselling Centre in Bangalore sharp by 6 PM, five days a week, and has been doing so for the past 36 years. Pankaja needs her assistant to hold her hands and walk her to her office room. Her patients see this and sometimes wonder how she does her work when she settles down in her chair. She gives them a beaming smile. It is clear that she values her work and looks forward to helping those who come to see her. She is credited with making Prasanna Counselling Centre one of the most trusted and sought after counselling centres in Bangalore under her leadership since 1980.[7]

The Prasanna Counselling Centre is situated in south Bengaluru at 20 km from my home in north Bengaluru. They charge a nominal fee of only Rs.2000/-. Theory class was from 6:00 to 8:00 PM every Tuesday and Friday. I drove my car for every class leaving home at 4:30 and returned at 9:30 PM. Theory class was for four months, and the practical classes were for two months. The practical class means observing the counselling sessions by our teacher Ms Pankaja Madam who counsels the help seekers coming to her for various issues. She was a high school teacher in Bengaluru, and after retirement at 58, she continues to keep her body fit even today.

Counselling means giving suggestions or advice to persons in distress to help themselves. It is a talking treatment for people facing problems such a family, marital, finance, job, society, education, depression, health, ethical and moral issues etc. It is done in a friendly manner without exercising any force, demand or compulsion. Both should have love and respect for each other.

The topics covered during the training course:

1) Bio-Psycho-Social development of an individual 2) Understanding normal and abnormal behaviour: Role of genetics, individual and environmental factors. Positive and negative emotions.3) Reactions to stress and stress-induced problems 4) Major mental problems 5) Tobacco, alcohol, drug abuse 6) sexual and marital problems 7) Age-specific mental health problems-child-adolescent. Middle and old age 8) Family, its role in individuals health and efficiency 9) Prevention of handicaps including mental handicaps 10) Promotion of health, life skills, positive mental and social health. 11) Individual-Family and society 12) Qualities of good counselling 13) Interviewing techniques and communicating skills 14) Steps in counselling and principles of counselling 15) Legal aspects of counselling 16) Life skills.

Prasanna Counselling Centre gets sincere teachers who work as a team without expecting any remuneration. Faculties were drawn from different disciplines who are experts in their field. My class strength was around 70, though, in the first week, it was nearly 100. The age group was from 18 to 72. Here also, I was the senior-most by age. The trainees were from different professions, including house makers, engineers, software professionals, college-going students, yoga teachers, etc. Of course, there were some four retired people like me also. It was an excellent experience to meet people from all walks of life of different age groups.

Role Models for Lifelong Learning:

I quote some senior citizens who continued to pursue studies or teaching.

1) Kochi: Karthyayani Amma tops the Kerala Literacy Mission exam at the age of 96:

In 2018 (b. 1922), Karthyayani Amma was selected as Commonwealth of Learning Goodwill Ambassador. Her learning methods and her story will now be seen in several publications across Commonwealth Countries. The aim is to spread awareness about distance education and open learning among 53 member nations of the Commonwealth. Karthyayani Amma, a school dropout at the age of 12, who hails from Multan, Alappuzha district in Kerala, used to work as domestic help. She scored 98 % in the "Aksharalakshmi (Million Letters)" literacy programme topped 4[th]standard equivalent exams for adults, and received a merit certificate. She also received Nari Shakti Puraskar Award from the President of India on March 8, 2020, on International Women's Day, a national award to recognise exceptional work for women empowerment. At 98, she travelled to Delhi by air for the first time to receive the award. Age is just a number. Incredible willpower, perseverance and quest to learn are important. She said, "If God wishes I would like to pass 10[th]exam and learn computers also". (Credit: Press reports)

2) Mangalore: Prof. Krishnananda Hegde receives PhD at 79 from Mangalore University. He completed his thesis in history in five years under a guide who is the same age as his son. Many people his age struggle with memory loss. He says, "Former Vice-Chancellor of Manipal University Dr. B.M.Hegde encouraged me to take up this course. PhD means passing through many hurdles. It helped me to keep my mind active, and I can remember everything. He was an Indian Information Service officer, retired from All India Radio, New Delhi, as Joint Director of news 20 years ago. (*Courtesy: Times Mirror, Bangalore February 16, 2014*).

3) Patna: At 95, Bihar man enrols for Master Degree. He is of an age few people reach, and there are more goals to be achieved, but 95- year Rajkumar Vaishya is still keen to fulfil his dream of acquiring a post-graduate degree and is working for it with help from his retired son and daughter-in-law. He has enrolled for a Master of Arts in Economics from the Nalanda Open University (NOU). "My aim is not to get a degree; the thrust is to study and gain knowledge of economics so as to understand the problems faced by the people and contribute something," says Vaishya, who retired in 1980 as a general manager in a private firm in Koderma(now Jharkhand).

Living in Patna after his wife's death with his second son and daughter-in-law, who also retired now, Vaishya said the academic atmosphere in the house helped him make up his mind to study further. His son Santosh Kumar in his early 70's retired from the National Institute of Technology, whereas his daughter-in-law retired as a professor from Patna University. "Initially, they told me studying is not an easy task at his age, but later agreed to support me in view of my commitment. My son will teach me mathematics and statistics and my daughter-in-law will pitch in with other help. I have decided to devote two hours daily in the morning and night to studies". Vaishya Said. NOU registrar says it was a pleasant experience for University Officials when told about Vaishya's keenness to join the post-graduate course. We enrolled him on September 8 for the 2015-16 session. He further said Vaishya's zeal was admirable, and the initiative sent out a positive message in society, particularly among senior citizens. NOU has also had a retired professor Ram Chandra Mishra Madhup, 84, registered for a PhD. Vaisya was born in Bareilly town in Uttara Pradesh in April 1920 and graduated from Agra University in 1938, and got a degree in law in 1940.

He regularly reads books, newspapers and magazines and watches TV serials. He can still read without spectacles and writes fluently in Hindi and English with a steady hand. He, however, uses a walker after fracturing his leg some years ago.

"Otherwise, I am healthy; the secret of my long life was simple living and leaving everything to God. I accept everything as it happens. Today tension kills more than anything else. "People, particularly the young, should learn to live without stress," Vaishya said. A vegetarian and lover of simple traditional Indian food he never consumed fried food. 'Overeating kills more people than starvation", he quipped. (*Courtesy: Times Mirror Bangalore September 15, 2015*)

4) Tokyo: A 96-year-old Japanese man Shigemi Hirata received his Guinness World Records certificate after earning a Bachelor of Arts from Kyoto University of Art and Design. Born in 1919, he is something of a celebrity on campus. After taking up pottery, Harita, a pensioner, took 11 years to complete his ceramic arts course. He said, "My goal is to live until I am 100". Harita, who served in the navy during World War II and has four great-grandchildren, added, "I am so happy. At my age it's fun to be able to learn new things". Japan's perky pensioners regularly set eye-popping records as the silver-haired generations enjoy long and healthy lives. Last year, 100-year -old Mieko Nagaoka became the world's first centenarian to complete a 1500 – metre freestyle swim. (*Courtesy: Times of India Bangalore, June 5, 2016*)

5) Udupi: At 94, teaching keeps his spirit high- For Tonse Kemmannu Srinivas Rao, teaching is not a passion but a way of life. He still wishes to teach students for a few hours, even today. Rao joined the profession in 1942 when he got appointed as a teacher at the Adi Udupi Government School. The school was established in 1986 and managed by his father, Sitaramayya. In 1947, Rao became headmaster. He retired in 1978, at the age of 55, but that did not stop him from continuing his service as a teacher. I am not happy with my physical condition, but it gives me great joy that I am still associated with children 38 years after retirement. Shankar Shetty, the present headmaster of the school, a former student of Rao, said, "He loved sharing knowledge with the children. Every Friday for three hours, he entertains students with the Mahabharata, Ramayana, Quran, and Bible stories. But

three years ago, he started developing a vocal disorder, due to which he could not speak loudly. But this did not weaken his spirit. He started using a notice board outside the classroom to write math problems. Students of any class were free to answer the questions or ask doubts. After 3 PM he would be present in front of the school office where teachers and students would approach him for guidance (*Courtesy: Times of India, Bangalore, September 21,2016*)

CHAPTER FIVE

Developing Hobbies

As we age, our immune system in the body reduces, and we are prone to stress even for small changes in our routine. Hence, it is necessary to strengthen our immune system, which helps to keep infections and cancers under control. The white blood cells are critical to these processes. Different kinds of white blood cells are made from our bone marrow. Some work to produce antibodies to fight bacteria and viruses, and some break down bacteria directly. Eating a balanced diet, sleeping and exercise help to fight illness. National Institute of Mental Health of the United States finds that routine stress can lead to serious health problems like heart diseases, high blood pressure, diabetes, other illnesses, and mental disorders like depression, anxiety, and loneliness. After retirement, people generally lose interest in the hobbies they loved once. In some cases, they lose contact with old friends. There are several opportunities to go out and mix with people of their age groups or youth.

After retirement, if we associate with some organisations, we can be active both physically and mentally. We have to go out from our home regularly to attend events organised by them. It is fascinating to note that studies show that seniors who care for pets enjoy reduced blood pressure and lower level of cholesterol. Pets are the source of companionship and joy. Here I quote the example of the United Kingdom. While the total population of the UK is 66.6 million, 50 per cent of UK adults own a pet. 26 per cent own 9.9 million dogs, 24 per cent own 10.9 million cats and 2 per cent own 900,000 rabbits. (*Source:*

https://www.pfma.org.uk/pet-population2019). Though licencing is not needed for most domestic pets, microchipping of pets is compulsory in the UK. It will reunite people with their lost or stolen pets, help tackle the growing problem of strays roaming the streets, and relieve the burden placed on animal charities and local authorities. Here I recollect my memory of 1991 when we had our first dog of Doberman breed. We purchased a pedigreed one-month-old puppy. I went to the shop along with my daughter, who selected one puppy who came to running to us when we looked to the cage. Later on, it turned out to be a female, and we named her 'Sheri'. She became a member of our family, giving love and affection to everybody. She was growing so fast within six months we could not manage, and then we drove her to our native place to be under the care of my relative.

I will name a few of the hobbies which we can take up after retirement. For instance: Gardening, Yoga practice, caring for the pet, reading theology, hiking, swimming, bicycling, indoor or outdoor sports, nature trekking, voluntary service, taking an active part in the resident welfare associations, farming, meditation, writing articles and books, cooking, bird - watching, travelling, fitness activities like joining a gym, studying genealogy, joining singing (*bhajana*) groups etc. Having a hobby can help us establish new connections, improve our mood and enhance our levels of coping with stress. Taking up hobbies and some occupation after retirement by seniors help them to lead a productive life. Thereby one can become a part of the community and get rid of boredom and isolation.

Here, I quote Mr Kini, 88, who provides voluntary service wearing a big Identity Card on his chest as 'Helping Hand' at M.S.Ramaiah multi-speciality hospital in north Bengaluru. He says, "I come here on my own vehicle by 9:00 AM sharp everyday 5 days a week and work up to 1:00 PM, and guide the patients to the respective wards based on their category of illness. I was a General Manager in a private company in Mumbai. I am hale and healthy even today after 30 years of retirement. I expect nothing from the hospital. I feel proud that I provide a service to the community and have a purpose of living."

Similarly, Mr Basavaraj, 79, who has opened a Xerox shop in a suburban locality in Bengaluru, says, "After retirement I wanted to be active instead of getting branded as retired. I set up this shop in my own building though I get sufficient income as rent for my living. I alone do all menial jobs related to Xeroxing like taking copies, stapling etc. I work morning and evening 3 hours each. I am happy that I need not worry how to pass the time." Many people like this kept busy and avoided age-related diseases.

As people age, health becomes a significant part of life. The National Health Service (NHS) UK says that most people aged 65 and above spend most of their time sitting and lying down. It means that such people are at high risk of lifestyle illnesses such as heart disease, obesity, diabetes, depression, hypertension and finally, early death. By remaining active and, healthy the elderly can fight back the ageing process.

Everyone agrees that keeping busy adds healthy years to one's life. After retirement, I also became a member of several organisations and societies to fill my calendar with many events and schedules. Interestingly, among them, two associations bear the name of youth. When I joined them, I felt that I would have been their member long back. Though sexagenarian, then I was admitted as a member of the following organisations. i) Youth Hostel Association of India (YHAI), Bengaluru Chapter ii) Youth Photographic Society (YPS), Bengaluru iii) Bird Watcher's Field Club, Bengaluru. It is benefitting me to lead a medicine-free life even today by associating with these professional groups. I came in contact with young and old who had their own business or job but joined these groups for their sheer passion for the activity. I always felt that I spent quality time while I attended offline or online events in these organisations.

1) Trekking -Wellness Walk: After retirement, I chose trekking as a new hobby which I did not even think about when I was young and more active. Trekking and walking may look like similar exercises on the face because the body mechanics are the same. But what happens inside of us during these two different activities-our muscles, joints and heart -is a world apart. While walking on flat terrain requires little effort-it is one foot in front of the other but walking on uneven terrain (trekking) is a dynamic workout where our heart rate and metabolic rate increase, causing calories to burn faster. Trekking strengthens our muscles by shifting our body weight, balancing our body and moving at different angles. It is also a weight-bearing exercise to build bone density.

Trekking is an outdoor adventure. It has different phases, say gentle walk on flat land and rugged terrain to mountain climbing and descending. It also provides a natural way to engage the core muscles in our torso and sharpen the body balance skills, which we do not get that type of lateral motion from walking on a treadmill or riding a bike. Trekking is an excellent mood booster because it combines the physiological benefits of exercise with the mental health benefits of being surrounded by nature and socialising with other people on the trail. Since technology gadgets also cannot be used during long trekking, the mind becomes very calm. Many studies have proved the link between the amount of time people spend in nature and their mental well-being. Some clinically proven benefits are reduction in stress and blood pressure, improved sleep and energy levels. Trekking is the ultimate cardio workout as it lowers the risk of heart diseases, decreases cholesterol, and helps control our weight.

Among different exercises for fitness, I liked trekking and walking for fitness. While walking, exercise is a daily routine which I describe later under the chapter-10, "Keeping preventive medicine six natural doctors" trekking is an annual event I undertake. While in service, I could not exercise regularly; however, after retirement, I concentrated on walking, looking for its many benefits to maintain good health. I started my annual event under the name of "Wellness Walk" since 2014, some with my people in the native place and others with YHAI.

1	Wellness Walk 2014 (July 18 to 27, 2014)	230 km, Bangalore to Tirupati-Tirumala Hills via Srivarumettlu route, Chittor District, Andhra Pradesh
2	Wellness Walk 2015 (October 23 to 25, 2015)	85 Kms, Sirsi to Varadahalli-Sagar, Shimoga District, Karnataka. Trek passes through dense forest.
3	Wellness Walk 2016 (April 14 to16 2017)	80 km, from Sirsi to Divgi via Yaana, Kumta, Uttara Kannada District, Karnataka. Nature created and carved a single rock of 120 feet perimeter and 90 feet height in Yaana. Prior permission from Forest Department is necessary.
4	Wellness Walk 2017 (November 11 to 12, 2017)	40 km, Yellapur to Ulavai, Dandeli, Uttara Kannada District. Trek route passes through dense reserve forest and perennial waterfalls. Prior permission from Forest Department is necessary.
5	Wellness Walk 2018 (January 24-27, 2019) with YHAI	70 Kms, Gerusoppa to Gokarn, Uttara Kannada District. Sharavathi River Boat Cruise 30kms and Beach trek 40 km from Honavar to Gokarna covering Baada Beach, Nirvana Beach, Paradise Beach, Half Moon Beach, Om beach, Kudle Beach.
6	Wellness Walk 2019 (November 07 -10, 2019) with YHAI	18 km, Kudremukh mountain Peak (to and fro distance) at an 1892 m above sea level. One has to take prior approval from the Forest department.
7	Wellness Walk 2020 (February 22, 2020)	18 km, Kodachadri mountain peak (to and fro distance), at an altitude of 1343 m above sea level, Shivamogga District a natural heritage site. (Solo trek). One has to take prior approval from the Forest department.

My published articles on some of the trekking experiences are presented below.

Wellness Walk 2014- Bangalore to Tirupati - Tirumala Hill :

I, at 67, undertook a long-distance walk of 230 km for the first time from Bangalore to Tirupati, followed by climbing 2400 steps to reach Lord Balaji Venkateshwara Shrine at Tirumala Hill. The trek took a journey of 10 days. I was among 200 trekkers, including people of all ages from 15 to 80 and all walks of life.

Why journey on foot? Shyam Mahindrakar says he regularly undertakes *padayatra* (trekking). "The walking always keeps one down to earth and keeps body, mind and soul with nature. Body toxins are removed due to heavy sweating, leading to no ailments for the next minimum one year. Not only confidence and stamina increase but also the body connects to spiritual power".

When Mr Narasimha Murthy, 35, a graphic designer and painter by profession, told during our casual discussion in October 2013 that he is undertaking *padayatra* to Tirumala Hills with family for the successive 9th year, my inner desire kindled. How I had developed a fascination for a journey on foot makes an exciting story. I saw a monk, 68th Jagadguru of Kanchi Kamakoti Peetham, who lived for 100 years, usually known as Paramacharya Mahaperiyava. His Holiness Chandrashekharendra Saraswati (May 20, 1894, to January 8, 1994) undertook several pilgrimages on foot. During one such visit to Karnataka, while passing from Hospet to Gadag, I had his *Darshana*, way back in 1979, when I was just 32, working as a young officer in a public sector bank in Koppal, Karnataka state and then the sage was 85 years old. I was pretty surprised to see him walking barefoot in the hot sun. A few disciples followed him, carrying necessary things in a cycle rickshaw.

Recently I searched Google and found out that in April 1978, His Holiness had undertaken a long six-year *padayatra* through Andhra Pradesh, Karnataka and Maharashtra and returned to Kanchipuram only in April 1984. He was installed as the head of the Mutt in 1907 at the age of 13. He continued for 87 years till his heavenly abode in 1994. He travelled the length and breadth of the country on foot. I wondered why he was undertaking such an enduring task, and I found him to be the simplest of the simple persons. His requirements concerning food, clothing and shelter etc., were minimum. At the same time, he was arranging to feed thousands of devotees in Kanchipuram who come to see daily *pooja,* but he used to take simple food. The places he used to stay were cattle sheds roadside, even sometimes near railway gates.

He walked around 12 km per day. The Google storey revealed that he had walked from Hubli to Dharwar at one stretch about 23 km. I found him as a person who lived a contented life and showed future generations that one can live in the simplest way to become a centenarian without greed and ego.

Mr Murthy told me that 10- day *padayatra* would be from July 18 to 27, 2014. I had several queries regarding the size and age of the group, dress code, footwear, stay, and food arrangements to complete this arduous journey successfully. The road distance from Bangalore to the foothill Tirupati-Srinivasa Mangapur was 230 km. Then we have to climb 2400 steps to reach the top of the Tirumala hills to have *the darshan* of Lord Venkateshwara Balaji. Further, *depending on the crowd,* we have to stand in a queue for nearly 5 to 10 hours before darshan. He suggested the following preparation materials: two yellow cotton *lungis,* two yellow veils, cotton *kurtas,* one white *lungi* and veil (to wear while taking Lord Balaji *darshan*), water bottle, torch, light-reflecting jacket to wear while walking in the night, comfortable walking shoes or slippers, cap, one-bed sheet, plastic mat or bedroll. As per the advice, I purchased all the trekking gadgets.

The distance of 230 km was to be covered in seven days. In other words, daily coverage ranged from 25 to 50 km. This distance factor terrified me. Running 68, I still doubted whether I would undertake *padayatra* and further; Mr Murthy said that if any health problem or accident happens, no other padayatri (trekker) will step back as they are under oath to reach Tirumala Hills. But the trip but organiser will arrange a taxi for home or hospital. I further understood that there would be two trucks, one for luggage and one for the cooks, along with ration. But finally, I decided to join the trip.

On July 18, 2014, wearing the newly purchased costume, I prayed at home in Bangalore. I started walking to reach Swami Veeranjaneya Temple near Hebbal flyover, about four km away. All *padayatris* assembled for the initiation ceremony to wear *Tulsi Mala* and sacred hand thread to make him *'Vritadhari'*. From

Bangalore, the *padayatra* passed through the following halting places viz. 1st day at Avalahalli (After 20kms); Kolar(45kms); Nangli(50kms); Mugli (35kms); Chittur(25kms); Pakalvaripalli(30kms); 7th day Srinivasa Mangapura(25kms). 8th day climbing steps to Tirumala Hills and halt and 9th day Lord Balaji *darshan* and halt,10th day return to Bangalore by bus. On the first day afternoon, we had sharing experience talk by senior padayatris, who regularly have been undertaking journeys for decades. I also shared my experience of how I got inspired by H.H.Mahapariyava, whom I happened to see in 1978. However, I am happy to realise my dream in 2014.

A typical day begins around 3 AM when the group starts walking. We are like a walking machine working from 3 AM to 9 PM with a brief interval for taking food. The purpose of wearing a reflector jacket is to signal the truck drivers, especially during the night, coming from the other direction on the highway as a precaution. We usually walked on the right side of the road. The pre-dawn walk is calm and pleasant, and during long-distance, we covered nearly 25 to 30 km before forenoon and 15 to 20 km in the afternoon. We usually sleep at schools, community halls and marriage halls for or most of the days. Devotees of Lord Balaji sponsored the breakfasts, lunches and dinners. Sometimes, local people extended hospitality on our journey, taking us to their house and offering tea and snacks.

The group consisted of around 200 people of both sexes from all walks, including medical professionals. Some ladies were walking barefoot, keeping a single water bottle on their heads. This *padayatra* gives an outstanding lesson to manage our life independently because it provides a unique experience to live with people from all income groups sections of the society for ten days. Though we were walking in a small group of 5-6 people of likeminded what I found was that the walking speed of each one differs. I used to cover around 3-4 km per hour as against 4-5 km by youngsters who always stayed ahead and could rest wayside under the trees, in schools and temples, but I had to walk without a break to keep pace with the whole group.

It also gives a lesson that we come to this world alone and also leave alone. No dear and near will come with us while leaving this materialistic world. Further, strong willpower is most important to complete the trekking journey. Since the breakfasts, lunches and dinners are scheduled in a fixed place well in advance in the accompanying truck, cooks would be waiting to serve food for you. If you are not able to reach on time, you will miss it. On the way, the local two-wheeler riders often offer lift, but we cannot accept because we would break the oath of moving on foot. If you have any ailment and require regular medicine and check-ups, you may not dare voluntarily take such endurance. You have to learn to live like an ordinary person because you cannot expect home comfort, whether for food, sleep, clothing, bathing, attending nature calls, etc. Sometimes we had to take baths in ponds or farm wells wayside in the open. You have to forget your status, position, past and future. You prepare for everything, and you only are responsible for anything unpleasant that happens on the way. But this endurance gives so much self-confidence at the end that you feel rejuvenated. Remember, it is not a stress test in the hospital but a real test in the field.

After 2014, every year till 2020, I led a wellness walk of 3 to 4 days along with youngsters to places covering around 40 to 80 km. However, in 2018, I joined the Sharavathy valley and beach trekking event organised by the Youth Hostel Association of India, Tumkuru chapter. This wellness walk raised my self-confidence and health status. The endurance we face during the journey keeps our bodies fit and motivates us to continue walking to stay fit. However, due to Covid-19 I had to discontinue my annual trekking and contend with daily brisk walking.

Wellness Walk 2015- Kadave to Shree Kshetra Varadapura Shreedharaasharma:

My Wellness Walk 2014, when narrated by me in my village Kadave, a small village situated at 10 km from Sirsi in Uttara Kannada District, 450 km north from Bangalore, created curiosity and interest among youngsters. My nephews and other relatives, who are relatively young, below 35, came to me especially to listen to my experience of pleasure & pain during the Tirupati journey. After clarifying doubts, so inspired that they insisted that I lead a short trek of 3 days covering 85 km from Kadave to Shree Kshetra Varadapura Shreedharaashrama in Sagar taluk of Shivamogga District. Varadahalli, also known as Varadapura, is a small village surrounded by picturesque location near Sagara town, Karnataka. The place is famous for the Samadhi of His Holiness Shri Shreedhar Swamiji, one of the great saints of the 20th century. Shreedhar Swami Maharaj was born on December 7, 1908, in Lad Chincholi, near Kalburgi in Karnataka. Every moment of his life was dedicated to the divine service before attaining heavenly abode Maha Samadhi on April 19, 1973, at his Varadapura hermitage.

Since it was a new experience for the youth, elaborate planning was necessary before undertaking the trek to Varadapura. Hence, a trial trip of one day made by car to prepare a travel schedule indicating the time & places for breakfast, lunch, dinner & halt, calculating the distance to be covered per day & required travel time. The excellent message of walking as printed handbills both Kannada & English were taken for distribution to the passer-by during the journey to create awareness on the health benefit of walking.

My faint memory goes back to the days of my childhood, probably when I was six years old (1953) when Shri Shreedhar Swamiji came to our newly started paddy processing mill at Umachagi, started by my grandfather. Then my grandfather performed *paadapooja* & served food to him in his open hands. Swamiji sprayed Holy water from his *Kamandalu* to all of us.

I had been to Haridwar during August 1972 and stayed at Shringeri Shankar Mutt. When the then branch manager of the Shringeri Shankar Mutt Shri. Annappa Manja came to know that I am from Sirsi. He asked me whether I could carry five litres of Holy *Ganga Jal*, which he will hand over to me in a sealed tin, to offer Shri Shreedhara Swamiji for his *Shravana Masa Pooja*, who was in the cave without giving *Darshana* to anybody. I learnt that he went to *ekanta,* solitary penance in the cave in 1967 itself. I went to Varadapura in September 1972 and handed over the *Ganga jal* to his disciple monk Sri Sachidananda Saraswati Swamiji. I had an opportunity to listen to the discourse of Shreedhar Swamiji in four languages, viz. Kannada, English, Marathi and Hindi through a loudspeaker. However, he was not giving *Darshana* to anybody. He gave discourses from inside the cave. The gist of his sermon was, "Why do you love this body so much which is made up of muscle & bones. This body is not permanent. During your days on this earth, travel on the path of truth & honesty". I always liked his simple lifestyle & the way he put his body to endurance. Many stories spoke of his spiritual powers, which I also got convinced through my own experience. During the Wellness Walk- 2015, there were about 20 participants and a pick-up van and car. The pick-up van had cooking gas cylinders, all ration & cooks to make food items. The car was to provide medical aid & attend emergencies if the need arises. The journey started from Kadave at 3.30 AM on the 1stday. The participants were from all walks of life, say, farmers, people in business, government officials etc. One Timmayya Hegde (52) had done padayatra from Kadave to Ganagapura, a *Dattapeetha* in Kalaburgi district 500 km as a barefoot solo walker, living on alms from the people on the way. He also travelled with us barefoot.

The first-day route was from Kadave-Sirsi-Siddapur, covering 52 km, after which everyone felt exhausted and expressed that they would not have fixed such a long distance of 52 km. The ideal length would have been only 30 km per day (18 km morning & 12 km afternoon), but the schedule was prepared without judging the walking capacity of newcomers. However, we reached Siddapur Shri Shankara Mutt, a temple with a marriage hall complex to stay at 10:30 PM. Since the cooks were with us, they had prepared the food well in advance, and we had a sumptuous dinner.

The second day started early morning at 4:00 AM as the padayatris had a bitter experience of walking in the scorching sun after 10.00 AM the previous day. On the roadside, people enjoyed juicy pineapple fresh fruit near Talguppa. Lunch was served at Shiravante Tripuranthakeshwara temple at 3:00 PM. Then we proceeded to Varadapura, which we reached late at 10:30 PM. On the way, we had dinner at Karkikoppa prepared by our cook at 9.00 PM. Some of us, including me, had a holy bath at Shreedhara Teertha before going to bed on the mattresses carried by us. Shreedhar Teertha is a perennial sacred water spring formed by Swamiji. No one knows the origin of water, and there is a pool constructed there to store the holy water. It is believed that this water will run with purity till the existence of the earth. It is also believed that this holy water has the medicinal power to cure skin-related diseases. The next day morning, after taking a bath at Shreedhara Teertha, we attended morning pooja.

Later, we attended pooja at noon. We also performed *Samoohika Padapooja* of Shri Shreedhara Paduke. We attended aarati & we had *Prasada Bhojana* (lunch). We had collected individual contributions from each participant to meet the expenses for the transport of luggage & hiring cooks. Then we donated whatever savings in cash and kind to Shreedharaashrama. On the way back near Talguppa railway station, we again enjoyed fresh juicy pineapple fruit along with chilli powder. Around 2:30 PM, we had a small meeting where everybody shared their two days experiences. On the third day, the family members of trekkers had also joined. So it was a wholesome relaxing, memorable experience for everybody strengthening self-confidence & good health.

Wellness Walk 2019-Kudremukha Peak:

A worthy life is a journey of adventures, challenges, discovery and service to others. Age is just a number, and keeping ourselves busy by engaging mentally, physically and socially is vital to make our life cheerful. Participation in trekking increases my self-confidence about my health and fitness. It keeps me away from the doctor. Tumkur unit of Youth Hostel Association of India (YHAI) organised the Kudremukha peak trek in November 2019. Kuduremukha is a small hill station near the Sahyadri mountain range of the Western Ghats region, about 20 kilometres from Kalasa inMudigere Taluk, Chikkamagaluru district, Karnataka state. I joined 70 members strong trek group, comprising people from all walks of life and age groups from 16 to 72. Surprisingly, I emerged as the senior-most trekker of the group. We made an overnight journey by bus from Bengaluru to Kudremukha town. This place once was buzzing with mining activities of Kudremukha Iron Ore Company Ltd, a Government of India enterprise. Its Head Office is in Bengaluru and pelletisation plant at Mangalore. It had an iron ore mine at Kudremukha, one of the world's largest iron ore mines, but it was closed in 2006 due to environmental issues. Thanks to Supreme Court, which declared Kudremukha as a National Park is one of the 16 most eco-sensitive biological hotspots in the world. The trek route covered 18 km distance (to and fro) to which participants took ranging from 8 to 11 hours.

Hence, Kudremukha town has now hundreds of doorless, roofless dilapidated vacant living quarters but beautiful rich bio-diversity treasure, lung space of the Mother Earth saved. Kudremukh in Kannada dialect "Kudre" means horse, and "Mukha" means face as Kudremukha peak appears like a face of a horse. Rolling green hills with descending fog and mist, the place makes serene, silent and beautiful. Moreover, the terrain was still moist due to the extended 2019 monsoon, which caused widespread floods in Karnataka. Kudremukh Peak is a paradise for trekkers and naturists, situated in the heart of the Chikmagalur District. Kudremukh trek is an adventure-filled journey. The scene from the Peak is breathtaking with the view of the skies and clouds over the Arabian Sea. One of the unique characteristics of this trek is the diverse landscapes that it offers en route, ranging from tall grass, shrubs and shola forests to gushing streams and rolling hills. The Peak is located in the

Kudremukh National Park, which is rich in flora and fauna. Kudremukha is the third-highest Peak (Altitude 1892 M) in Karnataka after Mullayyana Giri and Bababudanagiri. Kudremukha forest covers an area of 600 sq. km, with a variety of flora and fauna falling in one of the coffee hubs of Karnataka.

Our base camp was Kudremukha town at Padmavati Kalyana Mantapa. It gets spring water from the uphill forest. We had breakfast at our base camp. Then we travelled 6 km in a four-wheel-drive jeep to reach the forest rest house at Malladi, the starting point for trekking. This road amidst coffee plantations is very bumpy and not even asphalted.

We started our trek at 8:30 AM after getting instructions from Forest Officials to be always in a group and be back by 5:30 PM. Walking distance to the Peak is 9 km(one way) from Malladi. The landscape was interspersed with pockets of dense forests and meadows over vast stretches of green hills and valleys. The first hour was a path covered by tall grasses, crossing many streams filled with slippery rocks. Since rains recently receded, the leeches had a feast on us though we were equipped with eucalyptus sprays to ward off leeches. After a couple of hours, the climbing became very tough. The uphill trail was a zigzag, but the landscape was simply breath-taking as clouds kissing the hills. We reached the Peak by around 1 PM. It was pretty foggy with gusty winds at the Peak. But our mood was highly elated and got euphoric. The natural beauty, the panoramic view of hills and valleys and the feeling of conquering the Peak made us forget all our tiredness. Not only that, this endurance trekking was our own choice. We passed our body fitness test. Interestingly many of our fellow trekkers could not reach the top and returned halfway from *Ontimara* (Singletree), where people take a small break.

After taking lunch at the Peak, which we carried in our back-pack in the morning, we started descending at 2 PM. The landing was also a challenge as recent rainfall made the path very muddy and slippery. I felt the Kudremukha trek was the most beautiful and picturesque trek of the Western Ghats. We also came across lush green coffee, areca nut plantations, and many waterfalls. Since our organisers had taken permission from the Forest Department and paid the entry fees, the department also provided forest guides to accompany us. I counted that we traversed seven hills and six small streams. We returned to our base camp by 6:00 PM. Thank God everyone returned safely, and I felt I could join for next year's trek for a new place. The next day we went to Kurunjal peak (1160m), trailing 14 Kms (to and fro distance) in dense rainforest falling in the same Kudremukh National Park. On the third day, we visited Bhavi Konda and Somavathi enchanting waterfalls and returned to Bangaluru.

2) *Photography*:

I became a member of the Youth Photographic Society (YPS) Bengaluru.[1] Membership of the YPS has brought me close to many talented photographers in Bengaluru whose images have won prizes in several national and international exhibitions. The club has both experienced and amateur photographers as its members. Programmes are held every Saturday at 6:30 PM at YPS, State Youth Centre, Nrapatunga Road, Bengaluru. However, the outbreak of the Covid-19 pandemic resulted in having weekly meetings online at 5:30 PM through webinars attended from home. The activities of YPS continues as before uninterrupted. Photography experts talk on different fields like capturing photographs on birds, wildlife, advertising, fashion, travel, underwater, landscape, nature etc. YPS also brings out a monthly magazine, "Drishti".

Profile of members of YPS consists of software engineers, business people, journalists, homemakers. These photographers capture the beauty of nature's creation in the form of appealing images. They travel to less explored places in the pursuit of clicking photographs. These photographers love spending quality time in the tranquility of nature, waiting patiently hours together, risking their lives to click a particular moment. Which gets captions like 'Lion and lioness attacking wild beast', 'Birds in flight', 'Bird catches fish from inside the water', 'Python catches the prey'. Many amateurs bring their pictures, and seniors guide them on image, composition, lighting, subject, etc. They advise them how to click photographs more creatively.

The main advantage for me is to appreciate the work, enthusiasm, bravery of these young photographers. I am also thrilled by listening to their stories in capturing the photographs risking their life with wild animals like elephants, lions, tigers, pythons, etc. Though I cannot attempt such adventures at this age, I get a positive attitude by interacting with them.

3. Bird - watching:

My interest in bird - watching hobby started in 2015 at 68, when I returned from the United States with a binocular gifted by my daughter. Bird - watching is the best way to connect to nature for senior citizens. In November 2015, I visited the Ranganathittu bird sanctuary near Mysore, one of the finest and picturesque bird sanctuaries in India. This sanctuary hosts nearly 18000 birds during February every year, both Indian and migratory. One can see a variety of birds like cormorants, egrets, herons, storks, parakeets, ibis etc. While entering the bird sanctuary, adjacent to Dr. Salim Ali Interpretation Centre, I saw one big signboard which reads, "A tip for longevity: People say you can't make a living from bird - watching. That's perhaps true but, it is also true that man does not live by bread alone. Just look at the people who have no such hobbies and spend all the time solely on earning a living. After 60, when they retire from the official chair, they don't know what to do with all the time in their hands and just spend it watching the clock! If they had cultivated a hobby like bird - watching, perhaps they would have lived longer to enjoy their pension ---Dr. Salim Ali".

Dr. Salim Ali(1896-1987), one of the greatest ornithologists of all time, also known as 'Birdman of India', was the first Indian to conduct systematic bird surveys across India and authored several bird books. His whole life was out all the time walking in remote areas, looking for birds, listening in the company of birds, and never feeling alone. He was also the recipient of several national and international awards for his contribution to nature conservation.

After my first visit to Ranganathittu, I have visited several bird sanctuaries in Karnataka like Kokrebellur, Gudavi, Magadi, Attiveri and Mundigekere in Karnataka State. I also joined the birding informal voluntary group Bird Watcher's Field Club (BWFC) of Bangalore(bngbirds group), which has been in existence since 1972. The group organises bird walks, open to everyone, to different birding hotspots on the four Sundays of every month from 7:30 to 10:00 AM through bngbirds discussion e-group. The city's pleasant climate, number of lakes and gardens provide ample opportunity for birds to find food and shelter, and so the birders have been able to spot many species within the city and on the outskirts. With awareness regarding the conservation of nature, flora and fauna on social media, more and more people are attracted to these morning walks. Many amateurs, new photographers also join every month.

When we go out to watch birds, we also observe water, vegetation, and other animals, including reptiles. Such things rejuvenate our body, mind and soul. Medical professionals also agree that exposure to nature is necessary to reduce stress, restore mental power, health and happiness. Bird - watching combines several activities like walking, nature trekking, sun exposure, social networking, lifelong learning etc., the factors responsible for longevity. Bird - watching continues to grow in popularity among folks of all ages.

Fascinating facts of migratory birds:

Using a combination of the earth's magnetic field and the position of the sun and stars, the birds navigate a long-distance journey through 'Fly Ways'. Migratory birds connect our planet. World Migratory Bird Day (WMBD) is now celebrated twice a year, on the second Saturday in May and October.

1. The bar-headed goose- one of the world's highest-flying birds:

One of the most exciting things about the Bar-headed goose is its ability to fly over the Himalayas from its breeding ground in ground in Mangolia and China travel to its winter home in Asia. The bar-headed geese weigh about 2 to 3 kg. Around 7000 birds travel in batches of 50 to 500, fly from Mongolia to Magadi lake (Gadag district of Karnataka) every year to their winter home, some 5000 km distance crossing the tallest peaks of Himalayas. These birds fatten their body before flying, decrease their metabolic rate and chill their blood to maintain the hypoxic conditions for long-distance, high altitude (1000 M) flight. These birds are very friendly. I have seen them in the lake alongside ladies washing clothes and men bathing the cattle when visited Magadi Lake bird sanctuary.[2]

2. Alpine Swifts can fly for 200 days at a time, without landing:

Alpine Swifts are small birds weighing around 100 g. A combined team of researchers from Bern University and the Swiss Ornithological Institute has found that alpine swifts can fly for up to 200 days at a time without landing. To find out, the researchers attached very tiny sensors to six of the birds—the sensors measured light and acceleration. Though only three of the sensors were recovered when the birds returned, there was enough data to allow researchers to track their routes and whether they were flapping their wings or gliding. The birds in the study were captured in Switzerland and then released. Alpine swifts migrate to Africa and back every year. In analysing the data captured by the sensors, the researchers found that the test birds stayed in the air at one point for 200 days, covering approximately 10,000 kilometres in the process. The researchers' report, it is the longest flight duration ever recorded by a bird.[3]

3. Oriental Pratincole: Small but long-distance migrant birds:

Oriental Pratincole (OP) weighs about 60 to 100 gm. Research study on Oriental OP conducted by Australian Wader Studies Group (ASWG) and Tern Expedition Team of North-West Australia released fitted with a PTT (Platform Transmitter Terminal) some birds on March 4 2019. The satellite showed details of the location of the birds in different countries. The birds had reached the Central Island of Alamatti dam in Bagalkot district in Karnataka on April 22 2019, with a stop-over in Cambodia. Our BWFC's most respected member, who also worked Dr. Salim Ali, Dr. S Subramanya was requested by the Bombay Natural History Society (BNHS) in May 2019, to find out the bird and submit a report. Dr. Subramanya travelled from Bangalore to Bagalkot on May 12, 2019. He took the help from Karnataka State Forest Department. He found several nests of OPs, and most of them contained three eggs each at one spot. He saw some 25 nests being incubated. Since it is unethical to disturb the nesting process, he moved away after taking some photographs quickly. The tagged birds that Dr. Subramanya photographed, returned to Australia via Sri Lanka on December 20, 2019, making a return trip of 13000 km. They remained for 88 days on the breeding ground in the Bagalkot district. They left Bagalkot on July 14, 2019, for Sri Lanka.[4, 5]

Some of the most obvious questions that come to mind regarding the birds are: How do they eat and drink? When do they sleep? How do they get energy? It is revealed that they eat what is known as aerial plankton—a mix of fungus spores, small insects, seeds and even bacteria that float about in the sky. The water in their food is apparently enough to sustain the birds indefinitely. As for how and when they sleep, scientists are still divided. It is mind-blowing to think about how nature is supporting birds.

There are many lessons to learn from birds like following a leader, maintaining discipline, putting continuous efforts from birth to death, always keeping family and friends for strength and confidence. We wonder when we see ducks walking on the road following a strict lane discipline one behind another.

CHAPTER SIX

Organ and Body Donation

What happens to the body after death?

Nature is very efficient at breaking down human corpses. When we die, our heart stops pumping blood around our body, thus depriving our cells of oxygen, rapidly dying. Decomposing starts almost immediately, with the skin going through several changes in colour as the blood stops circulating, leaving the body an ash colour. However, different cells die at different rates. For example, brain cells die within a few minutes, while skin cells survive over 24 hours after death. Rigor mortis occurs soon after death. A few hours after a person dies, the body's joints stiffen and become locked in place. This stiffening is called rigor mortis. Depending on body temperature and other conditions, rigor mortis lasts approximately 24 hours depending upon ambient temperature. The phenomenon is caused by the skeletal muscles partially contracting. Sometimes the survivors of the dead value the traditional funeral, burial and cemetery plot over whole body donation. They want to visit their loved ones at the cemetery. When we give serious thought, we realise that burning our bodies to ashes or burying them to decay in a graveyard has no meaning. Then why not donate this body and tissues for a good cause.

Our life is precious, but it is not permanent. So organs and tissues are gifted to needy people who can lead a happy life after having transplanted into their bodies. It also provides an unparalleled opportunity to give someone a second life. Our donation impacts not only the life of one person or family but also overall help for society as a whole. It is also one way to be alive after death. One may want to donate organs and also the whole body. Yes! That's possible, but after their death. Doctors can remove donated organs first and then coordinate body donation with the anatomy department. That is what exactly I did for my body. I became a body donor and also an eye donor at 68. I am writing more details on the topic to make some readers decide for the noble cause. With medical advances, it is now possible to use retrieved organs and tissues to enhance the life chances of those suffering from a range of terminal conditions such as renal, liver and heart failure.

Moreover, the people suffering from these conditions are on the rise. Many people ask the question of whether 70 + persons can donate eyes. There is no age bar for eye donation, provided the person is free from significant ailments. Even those people who have undergone cataract surgery of both eyes can also donate. Only the cornea is taken out, which is a tissue intact even after the cataract surgery.

Organ Donation involves surgically removing an organ from one person (donor) and transplant it into another (recipient) whose organ has failed or been damaged. A solid organ is our Heart, Lungs, Kidney, Liver, Pancreas, Intestine etc. Tissue is a group of cells performing a particular role in the human body like the eye's cornea, bone, skin, heart valve, blood vessels, nerves and tendons, etc. The age limit for organ donation varies, depending upon whether it is a living donation or cadaver (brain dead human body) donation. However, for most organs, the deciding factor is the person's physical condition and not age. Specialist healthcare professionals decide which organs are suitable on case to case basis. There are two types of organ donation.

Living Donor Organ Donation: A person during his life can donate one kidney (the other kidney is capable of maintaining the body functions adequately for the donor). A portion of the pancreas (half of the pancreas is adequate for sustaining pancreatic functions) and a part of the liver (the liver segments will regenerate after a while in both recipient and donor).

Generally, a donor must be more than 18 years old and should approve organ removal.

Deceased Donor Organ Donation: A person can donate multiple organs and tissues after (brain-stem/cardiac) death. Anyone, regardless of age, race can contribute. One donor can save life up to eight lives. What matters is the health and the condition of the organ when we die. Organs and tissue from people in their 70s and 80s have been transplanted successfully all over the world. To date, the oldest deceased donor in the U.S. was age 93. A deceased donor can generally donate the Organs & Tissues with the age limit of Kidneys and liver: up to 70 years, Heart and lungs: up to 50 years, Pancreas and Intestine: up to 60-65 years, Corneas and skin: up to 100 years, Heart valves: up-to 50 years, Bone: up-to 70 years. Donated whole bodies are primarily used for medical education and research. They are used for gross anatomy, surgical anatomy and further medical education and research.

The time frame for transplant: Doctors have to be quick as there is a time limit for transplant after the harvest of the organ, say Heart and Lungs 4-6 hours, Intestine 6-10 hours, Liver 12-15 hours, Pancreas 12-24 hours and kidney 24-48 hours. Decisions should be quick for both donors and recipients.

One can be a donor by expressing one's wish in the authorised form for organ and tissue donation at local medical colleges with transplanting facilities. I became a body donor for M.S.R. medical School in Bangalore. Sometimes it so happens that even though someone is pre-registered, the transplant organisation finds out years later that they passed away. Unfortunately, the donor never expressed their wishes to the family members.

Present Scenario of Organ transplant:

In India, there is a growing need for organ and tissue transplantation due to a large number of organ failures. Though there is no organised data available for the required organs, the numbers are estimated at 500 000 due to the non-availability of organs. Every year, a number of patients requiring kidney stand at 200 000, liver patients at 200 000, heart patients at 50 000 and eye corneas at 100 000. Ideally, India should collect 200 000 corneas a year as only 50-60 % could be utilised to give vision to one lakh people in need of it. Along with harvesting corneas, blood samples of the corpse for conducting tests to check for infections. In the case of disease, corneas cannot be used for transplant. It is reported that there are 300-400 deaths in Bangalore every day, but hospitals get only 15 cadaver eye donations. Only a few people die in circumstances where they can donate their organs. That is why we need people to take a pledge for Organ Donation and register themselves as potential Donors. There is a vast gap between demand and supply for transplant.[1, 2, 3]

The first organ transplant was conducted in the 1970s in India (it was a kidney transplant). India has made a few strides forward since then, but a lot more needs to be done. The number of transplants done annually has been gradually rising. Around 6000 kidneys, 1500 livers, and around 500 hearts and 25000 eyes are transplanted annually in India.There is a poor rate of deceased organ donors in India: 0.52 per million population(pmp) compared to some of the better performing countries such as U.S.A. 38.0, Spain 37.9, Estonia 24.8, Portugal 24.6 (Source 2020: http://www.irodat.org). Living organ donors rate: India 7.74, pmp against South Korea 49.74, Turkey 41.15, Israel 31.7, Iceland 23.33. India is struggling with an acute shortage of organs for transplantation. At least 15 patients die every day waiting for organs, and every 10 minutes, a new name is added to this waiting list. Awareness of organ donation is, therefore, the only way out of this depressing scenario. If there are more potential donors, the likelihood of organs becoming available to save lives would be more.

Key facts about laws governing organ donation in some major countries:

Singapore: The city state's organ donor policy assumes all citizens above 21 are willing donors unless they have registered with the Government that they wish to opt-out. It is known as "presumed consent".

European Union: Many European countries, including Austria, Belgium, Denmark, France, Italy, Greece, Norway, Switzerland, Spain, and Sweden, have laws similar to Singapore's 'presumed consent legislation. Here the eyes of the dead belong to Government. If a person wants to opt out, they have to make a will to the effect that their corneas must not be harvested. In most of these countries, family consent is also sought. The Government's goal is to achieve zero corneal blindness in their countries. Organ transplants are carried out free of cost under the Public Health System.

United States: Organ donation in the United States is based on the "informed consent" principle. Under the 'informed consent,' individuals must consciously decide to donate organs after death and indicate their willingness to do so.

Japan: Both the potential donor and the family must consent to establish 'brain death' as well as organ transplantation. The donor card must be signed by the potential donor and two witnesses, including a close relative. The family has the right to withdraw consent to donate at any time. Our country also adopts the policy of "informed consent". Either prior registration for donating the body or approval after the death by the survivors for donating the body and organs are necessary.[4]

Road traffic accidents and intracranial haemorrhage (bleeding in the brain) are the two leading causes of brain death. They are the source of cadaveric organic donations. The youth are mainly involved in road traffic accidents, while the elderly suffer bleeds. In the United States, the primary source of organs for transplant is victims of road accidents (nearly 85%). But in India, the figure is abysmally low despite having the highest rate of road accidents in the world. That is because most do not pledge their organs. Many believe in the theories of rebirth and are opposed to the thought of sending out a mutilated body to burn or bury. The total number of brain deaths due to accidents is nearly 1.5 lakhs annually in India. Other causes of brain death such as Intra Cerebral Hemorrhage (ICH)-I.C. bleed and brain tumours would potentially add more numbers. There is a need for two lakh kidneys, 50,000 hearts, 50,000 livers and 100000 eye corneas for transplantation every year. Even if 5 to 10 per cent of all brain deaths are appropriately harvested for organ donation, technically, there would be no requirement for a living person to donate organs. However, organ utilisation has improved dramatically with the National Organ and Tissue Transplant Organization (NOTTO). The distribution Pan India is much better with much less wastage. The cost of a transplant for a kidney is Rs.3 lakhs, heart and liver Rs.12 lakhs each while for corneal transplant ranging from Rs.50000 to 100000. With the launch of eye banks, a corneal transplant is free for poor patients.

Life after organ transplant:

An organ transplant, especially kidney, liver and heart, is often seen as the second inning in life for those receiving it from healthy donors. But living with a foreign body is not as simple as it seems. In most cases, organ recipients have to depend on expensive immune-suppressants or anti-rejection drugs all their lives to boost resistance. They should be careful with their diet and dosage of medicines and watch out for any side effects caused by long term intake of steroids. Recipients have to lead a highly disciplined life concerning taking tablets, diet, exercise and sleep. The cost of drugs is also very high ranging from Rs.10000 to 15000 per month. However, a transplant is easy on the eye. A corneal transplant is a journey from darkness to light. It is the most visible transformation for a person suffering from cornea damage by birth or by accident. Unlike other organs, the donor's corneas need not match the recipient's since the cornea is tissue, not an organ. Usually, a young person's cornea is transplanted to another young person in need to live longer. Here the aftercare cost is also less, maybe around Rs.1000 per month only on eye drops.

Transplant process:

While organ donation for therapeutic purposes is covered under the Transplantation of Human Organs Act (THOA 1994), a whole-body gift is covered by the Anatomy Act 1984. Organ and Tissue donation is defined as giving life to others after death by donating their organs to the needy suffering from end-stage organ failure.

Body donation is defined as giving one's body after death for medical research and education. Those donated cadavers remain a principal teaching tool for anatomists and medical educators teaching gross anatomy. If there has been a post-mortem examination, bodies are not accepted for teaching purposes. However, if only the corneas are to be donated, a body can be left for research.

Every Registered Transplant hospital has a Transplant Coordinator under the Transplantation of Human Organ Act to coordinate all matters relating to removal or transplantation of Human Organs or Tissues or both and assist the authority to remove human organs. Though their work is more related to deceased organ donation, they are also responsible for living organ donation. The patient can register for inclusion in the waiting list through a registered transplant hospital. Every patient who has developed end-stage organ failure may not be fit for an organ transplant. The treating physician of the hospital shall make an evaluation and decide if the patient needs a transplant and meets the criteria to be listed. Like kidney transplants, other than the blood group, the main criteria are time since the patient is on regular dialysis. Similarly, for other organs, standards are different based on medical history, the current condition of health, and other factors.

There is a waiting list of people waiting for receiving an organ. Every patient who has developed end-stage organ failure may not be fit for an organ transplant. The patient can register for inclusion in the waiting list through a registered transplant hospital. The treating physician of the hospital shall decide if the patient needs a transplant and meets the criteria to be listed. Like kidney transplants, other than the blood group, the main criteria are the time since the patient is on regular dialysis. Similarly, for other organs, standards are different based on medical history, the current condition of health, and other factors.

Once you are added to the national organ transplant waiting list, you may receive an organ on the same day, or you may have to wait many years. It depends on how well you match with the donor, how sick you are, and how many donors are available in your local area compared to the number of patients waiting.

There is a massive gap between demand and supply for transplants. More patients require different organs than the number of organs available for transplantation. That is why there is an urgent need to create awareness about organ donation. More people decide to take the pledge and donate organs to reduce the waiting list number. In Cadaver Organ Donation Programme, confidentiality is always maintained, unlike living donors who usually already know each other. The protocol for organ distribution is the state priority. If no match is found, they are offered regionally and then nationally until a recipient is located. Every attempt is made to utilise donor organs. The National Organ and Tissue Transplant Organization (NOTTO) operates the waiting list and organ allocation system.

NOTTO maintains a waiting list of patients needing transplantation in terms of the following:- Hospital wise, organ wise, Blood group-wise, patient age, urgency (on a ventilator, can wait etc.), Seniority in the waitlist (First in, First Out).

Recently the Government has tweaked organ donation criteria. A hospital with a brain dead patient can retrieve organs and transplant them to patients undergoing treatment at the same facility (press report August 30, 2020).

The most common organ donated by a living person is a kidney, as a healthy person can lead a completely normal life with only one functional kidney. Kidneys transplanted from living donors have a better chance of long-term survival than those transplanted from a deceased donor. Nearly 90% of all kidney transplants currently in India are from a living donor.

In addition to the kidney, part of the liver, lung and, small bowel can be donated and transplanted. For all forms of living donor transplants, the risk to the donor must be considered very carefully. Before a living donor transplant can go ahead, there are strict regulations to meet and a thorough process of assessment and discussion.

As per the TOHA, 1994 Brain Stem Death is legally accepted as death. A brain stem dead person cannot breathe on his own; however, the heart has an inbuilt mechanism for pumping as long as it has a supply of oxygen and blood. A ventilator continues to blow air into the lungs of brain stem dead persons. Their heart continues to receive oxygenated blood, and medicine is given to maintain their blood pressure. The heart will continue to beat for a while after brain stem death - this does not mean that the person is alive or that there is any chance of recovery. Brain death is not the same as a coma. People can recover from a coma but not from brain death.

Donor's vital organs will be transplanted into those individuals who need them most urgently. Gifts of life (Organs) should match the recipients based on medical suitability, the urgency of transplant, duration on the waiting list and geographical location. NOTTO and its state units (Regional Organ and Tissue Transplant Organization-ROTTO & State Organ and Tissue Transplant organisation- SOTTO) will work round the clock, every day of the year and cover the whole country. Tissue is occasionally matched, e.g. for size and tissue type, but otherwise is freely available to any patient needing a transplant.

When a person is declared a brain stem dead in the hospital, they are immediately put on a ventilator and other life support systems. After the death at home, only eyes and some tissues can be removed. Solid-organ donation (heart, lungs, liver, pancreas, kidneys) requires blood circulation to maintain these organs until retrieval. It is possible in brain-stem death where the functioning of these organs can be supported for some time. However, organs after cardiac death can also be harvested, provided the time gap is minimal.[5]

Legal & Ethical Issues:

The Central Government has established NOTTO, which has five Regional Networks ROTTO. They develop SOTTO (State Organ and Tissue Transplant Organisation) in every State/U.T. SOTTO functions in every state. U.T. NOTTO maintains the national registry for organ donation & transplant. They keep 1) Organ Transplant Registry 2) Organ Donation Registry 3) Tissue Registry 4) Organ Donor Pledge Registry. As per the THOA Act, buying/ selling of organs in any way is punishable and has significant financial and judicial punishment. In India and any part of the world, selling an organ is not permissible.[6]

Organ Donation and Religion:

All major religions support organ donation as an individual right and encourage it as an act of generosity and compassion. It is very noble to donate the organs of our bodies. It helps the survival of another human who will cherish their life.

Hinduism: Organ donation is giving an organ to help someone who needs a transplant. Many references support organ donation in Hindu scriptures. Daana is the original word in Sanskrit for gift, meaning selfless giving. It is also third in the list of the ten Niyamas (virtuous acts). Life after death is a strong belief of Hindus and is an ongoing process of rebirth. The law of Karma decides which way the soul will go in the next life. "As a person puts on new garments giving up the old ones, the soul similarly accepts new material bodies giving up the old and useless ones." Bhagavad Gita, chapter 2:22. Scientific and medical treatises (Charaka and Sushruta Samhita) form an important part of the Vedas. Sage Charaka deals with internal medicine, while Sage Sushruta includes features of organ and limb transplants.

Jainism: For Jains, after death, the soul departs, and the body is of no use to anyone and therefore donating organs of your body to other human life will mean doing a great deed on your part. The Jain community considers eye donation a sublime form of charity and believes in a strong link between 'daan' (charity) and 'moksha' (salvation).

Sikhism: The Sikh philosophy and teachings support the importance of giving and putting others before oneself. Seva (the act of selfless service, to give without seeking reward or recognition) is at the core of being a Sikh. Service can also be about donating your organ to another. Sikhism does not attach taboos to organ donation and transplantation and stresses that saving a human life is one of the noblest things you can do. The Sikh religion teaches that life continues after death in the soul and not the physical body. The last act of giving and helping others through organ donation is consistent with and in the spirit of Sikh teachings.

Catholicism: Organ, eye, and tissue donation is considered an act of charity and love, and transplants are morally and ethically acceptable to the Vatican. (Pope John Paul II, Evangelium Vitae, no. 86)

Islam: The Fourth Conference of the Islamic Fiqh Council determined that organ transplantation offers "clear positive results" if practised "...to achieve the aims of sharee'ah . This concept tries to achieve all that is good in the best interests of individuals and societies to promote cooperation, compassion and selflessness." Provided that "shar'i guidelines and controls that protect human dignity" are met, "It is permissible to transplant an organ from a dead person to a living person whose life or basic essential functions depend on that organ, subject to the condition that permission be given by the deceased before his death, or by his heirs after his death...." Regarding living donation, it is permissible to transplant organs such as a kidney and or a lung "in order to keep the beneficiary alive or to keep some essential or basic function of his body working." (Resolutions of Islamic Fiqh Council of the Organization of the Islamic Conference, Fourth Conference, Jeddah, Kingdom of Saudi Arabia, 18-23 Safar 1408 AH/6-11 February 1988 C.E.).

Judaism: In principle, Judaism sanctions and encourages organ, eye, and tissue donation to save lives. According to Rabbi Elliott N. Dorff, Professor, American Jewish University, Chair of the Conservative Movement's Committee on Jewish Law and Standards, saving a life through organ donation supersedes the treatment of a dead body. Transplantation does not desecrate a body or show a lack of respect for the dead. Any delay in burial to facilitate organ donation is respectful of the decedent. Organ donation saves lives and honours the deceased. The Conservative Movement's Committee on Jewish Laws and Standards has stated that organ donations after death represent not only an act of kindness but are also a "commanded obligation" that saves human lives. (On Educating Conservative Jews Regarding Organ Donations, May 1996). [7]

Probably there is nothing more unfortunate than the inability to avert a preventable fatality in life. It is estimated that more than a million people suffer from end-stage organ failure. Organ transplantation is the medical procedure that could have saved them giving them a second lease of life. August 13 is celebrated as 'World Organ Donation Day' and is dedicated to motivating people to pledge to donate their organs. Organ donation is probably the noblest way to live beyond one's death and giving another person a new lease of life. Do bear in mind that no one is too old or young to be a donor, as anyone above 18 years can pledge to donate their organs.

Despite being the second-most populous nation in the world, the organ donation rate in India is one of the lowest globally. Significantly few people are opting to donate their organs. While over the last five to six years, there has been an increase in the number of donors, yet as the base is tiny, the impact is relatively low. In particular, the southern state of Tamil Nadu has been aggressively promoting and supporting the cause of organ donation. It was the first state in India that made the declaration of brain death mandatory. Alongside whenever needed, citizens, traffic police and government bodies come together in a concerted manner to create green corridors. Special routes enable harvested organs to reach the intended hospital waiting for it as quickly as possible.

Organ donation is one of the greatest medical marvels of the twentieth century, which has saved the lives of several patients. The disparity between the enormous demands for the organs and their poor supply is the main issue. Our country's total organ donation shortage can be met even if only a few victims of fatal accidents serve as organ donors. Organ donation and successful retrieval of lifesaving organs are complex processes involving the coordination of multiple transplant teams.

Concept of Body Donation at M.S.Ramaiah (M.S.R.) Medical College, Bengaluru: The mortal remains of human beings are of no use when we burn or bury them. The quality of doctors graduating from medical schools needs a strong foundation and learning of the human system, which can be assured only by the experience of cadaver dissection. Advances in surgical skills such as laparoscopy, neurosurgery and vascular surgery need periodic practice mechanisms. Towards this objective premier medical science institutions establish "Cadaver Banks". Adopting the concept of "Live Well and Leave Well," we could immensely contribute to society for the cause.

M.S.R. Medical College, which got pledge by a body donor, provides free transport service within the city of Bangalore and also about 50 km radius to shift the body. However, if death occurs in a place that requires travelling of more than 6 hours, it does not serve the purpose. In that case, they coordinate with the local medical colleges. Just one can call medical college 24x7 helpline casualty service, which sends an ambulance to shift the body. The body is stored in cold storage first, and the following day cadaver would be moved to the morgue. After the donor body reaches the Department of Anatomy, a body receipt form will be given from the department. The receipt can be used to get the death certificate from the corporation. Around 80 million people need a transplant. Everybody, even up to age 90, can give the body. The health of the organ is important than age. Suppose the death is due to a natural cause. In that case, organ donation consists of only eyes, heart valves, ligaments, tendons and skin for the transplant. However, suppose there is brain death when the heart is still functioning. In that case, the organs such as the heart, kidney, pancreases and liver can be used for transplant with the written consent from close relatives.

When I decided to donate my body for medical science education and research, I rushed to M.S.Ramaiah Medical College, near my house in North Bangalore. The Helping Hand at the reception directed me to Anatomy Department. The Doctor-In Charge told me that I could pledge to donate both my whole body and eyes. She handed me two blank forms to fill. I returned duly filled with two passport-sized photographs, signed by me, witnesses my wife and daughter. My friend who had a cataract eye operation requested me to inquire whether he could donate his eyes. The doctor said that even the cataract operated people who are in good health can donate their eyes. Subsequently, I again went to the hospital.

I submitted a duly filled form after having my wife's signature as a witness on the body pledge form and my daughter's signature on the eye cornea pledge form. Later, the body donor Identity Card and the eye donor Identity Card came to my house through a courier. My wallet always contains these cards because I do not know when, where, and what death comes through. My wishful thinking is that peaceful death should come either during sleep or in full cheerfulness without being admitted to the hospital. Once admitted to the hospital, I know I will be identified mainly by patient number, and my name will be secondary. Dead means for some period only. Then I am remembered only anniversaries. The most significant benefit of donating the body and organ while still alive is the feel-good factor for the mind and pride to be helpful for a good cause even after death. It impacts our health too. The doctor at the medical college told me that after handing over the body, no part is given back to the kith and kin for the last rituals except hair. Since I have thin hair on the head, I do not think our people will get anything back! I put this chapter to create awareness of how important to decide to pledge to gift the body and organs when we are alive because 80 million people are currently waiting for an organ transplant in India.

After my death, my corpse would be utilised to further medical science research, a continuous human welfare process. If death comes home, my people have to telephone the M.S.R. medical college, and they will send the ambulance. But before taking the body, they require a death certificate issued by a Registered Medical Practitioner who has to indicate the cause of death. This certificate is essential to complete the process of body donation. When the deceased person's survivors are in grief, sometimes body donation will become a secondary issue. Of course, I made a lamination for my body donor I.D. Cards and kept in my pouch. My people also need not search for the telephone number to contact the hospital.

Since I am also an eye donor, my body is first taken to the ophthalmology department to remove my eye corneas. Then the corpse would be handed over to the anatomy department for medical education and research. The body will be in the morgue. The carcass is used by medical scientists, physicians and other scientists to study anatomy, identify disease sites, determine the causes of the death and provide tissue to repair a defect in a living human being. Dissecting a human body is essential for training aspiring physicians. Lifeless bodies become lifesaving tools. While organ donation is a point of pride but it is stigmatised. Most people have only a vague notion of what 'body donation" means. While a donated organ can save a life, a body provides the foundation to save many more. In most medical Colleges, for the sake of hands-on learning, they allot one cadaver (dead human body) to every four to six students. Besides this, the Physician Assistant and Nurse Practitioner course also require corpses.

Since senior citizens can donate eyes along with dead bodies, some more facts are described here. Sex, age, religion, wearing spectacles, diabetes, or any bodily illness are absolutely no bar for eye donation. One should close the eyelids immediately and put a wet cloth on both eyes. Keep the eyes on the forehead, raise the head with a pillow and put off the fan and switch on the air conditioner if available. Eyes have to be harvested within six hours of death. Removal of eyes will not disfigure the face of the departed as eyelids are closed skillfully. Removal of eyes takes only about 20-25 minutes. Since the cornea is a tissue, entire eyeballs are not removed but only the top layer during eye donation. A blood sample of the dead body is also taken to check for any infection.

Many times pledging of body or organs does not translate into donation after death. The main reason is the lack of awareness among the family members and the institution not having the necessary infrastructure to carry out the harvest. Pledging does not help donation of a body or eye happens only after death.

Concessions offered to body donors by M.S.R. Medical College:

Annual free Master Health check-up is offered for those donors who have registered. It includes general check-ups and basic investigations. Like complete haemogram, blood grouping and Rh typing, blood sugar fasting, lipid profile, blood urea, creatinine, urine routine, total protein/SGOT/SGPT, E.C.G., Chest X-ray(P.A.) and physical examination and advice by the physician(Diet advice if required). Annual free Ayurvedic massage at Gokula Ayush Arogyadhama. Besides above 50% concession for clinical services, investigation, and treatment charges at M.S.Ramaiah Medical Teaching Hospital, Gokula Ayush Arogyadhama and Pranic Healing Department.

However, I have not availed of any of these services so far. Thank God. My theory is as long as I have no health issues, why should I go for such a check-up? You may find it an extreme case because everybody says after 60, one should go annual body check-up. When trekking every year to the peaks, hills, walkathons with youngsters, my self-confidence says I am physically and mentally fit. If at all any complications arise, anyway test has to be taken. My routine walking, food discipline and sleep discipline has instilled this much confidence in my body fitness. M.S.R. Medical College also organises an annual event, 'Abhinandan', the Body Donor's Day, to express gratitude to the body donors who are nearly 3500 now. If I am in town, I will attend. There will be expert talks by specialists on preventing diseases generally faced by senior citizens in old age. The M.S.R. Medical College also hosts a sumptuous buffet lunch after the function, which was similar to nothing less than a marriage lunch. The body donor's also sharing their views on fitness and health during old age.

Organisations promoting organ donation movement in India:

They are creating public awareness of the need for organ donations – especially those from living donors. They are helping people to get transplants enabling them to enjoy a more active and independent life. Excellent work contributes to the education and training of the people, taking care of organ needing patients to attain superior quality treatment. Though there are many, only a few are listed here below.

Chennai: Multi-Organ Harvesting Aid Network (MOHAN), MOHAN Foundation, offers an online "Ambassador Training on Organ Donation" certificate course for those interested in organ transplant promotion. The topic covers the present status of organ donation, vital organs needed by the patients, deceased and live organ donors, legal and ethical issues etc. The coaching is through videos, medical expert talks, workshops and interactive webinars with transplant surgeons. I have also undergone this helpful training. (https://www.mohanfoundation.org/); Mumbai: National Kidney Foundation India(http://www.nkfi.in/), Narmada Kidney Foundation (http://www.narmadakidney.org/); Bangalore: Bangalore Kidney Foundation (B.K.F.) (https://www.bkfindia.in/), Gift Your Organ Foundation (www.giftyourorgan.org), The Jeeva Sarthakathe (http://www.jeevasarthakathe.karnataka.gov.in/), Dr. Rajkumar Eye Bank, (https://www.narayananethralaya.org/eye-bank/);

Hyderabad: Eye Bank Association of India (https://www.ebai.org/); Delhi: Parashar Foundation (https://www.organindia.org/).

Stories of Role Models for organ Donation:

1) Hyderabad: *Dead man gives a new lease of life to seven*: Seven people waiting for organ transplant got a fresh lease of life on Tuesday when the family of K.Venugopal, a security officer at a jewellery store, declared brain-dead, donated his organs.

People waiting for kidneys and liver for over two years were beneficiaries of the 30-year old's precious organs. A resident of Uppal, Venugopal, was going on a two-wheeler to his father-in-law's house at Nagarjuna Sagaron on April 10 to spend the weekend with his wife. A speeding car coming from the opposite direction hit him. Venugopal, who was not wearing a helmet, was thrown off his vehicle, and he suffered critical head injuries. He was rushed to the nearby Kamineni Hospital at LB Nagar. His family members said that though he battled for life in the I.C.U. for two days, he was declared brain-dead on April 12. He is survived by his wife and 15-month old son Jeevan. His liver was transplanted in a 50 year –an older man suffering from hepatitis infection for two and a half years. His kidneys saved a 35 older woman, a patient of chronic renal failure. She had been on dialysis for the previous three years. Both the transplants were done at Kamineni Hospital, which facilitated retrieval of his organs in coordination with the Mohan Foundation. Another kidney was transplanted in a 47-year older man who had been on dialysis for the last three and half years at Global Hospital. Transplant surgeons at these hospitals said that all the receivers were stable. Venugopal's heart valves were sent to Innova Hospital and eyes to L V Prasad Eye Hospital. Although the family was in deep shock, they were happy that he would live in seven others. Venugopal's wife, Swapna, and the other family members wasted no time giving consent to donate his organs. Venugopal's cousin Ganesh remembers him as a highly energetic and helpful person." Venu helped several people when he was alive and now he is helping others in death too." Said Ganesh. (Credit: Times of India April 14, 2010)

2) Hyderabad: *Mo's Organs give a new lease of life to two*: 69-year-old noted poet V.V.Mohan Prasad, also known as 'Mo', suffered a massive brain haemorrhage in August 2011, resulting in paralysis was rushed to the Sumukha hospital, Vijayawada. The doctors informed the family members his chances of survival were slim. When his heart was also failing to respond to the treatment, the doctors declared him brain dead. Since Prasad's last wish to donate his organs to the needy, he was immediately put on a ventilator until organ separators arrived. On August 2, the family members consent to donate his organs to give life to as many as possible. His kidneys, liver, eyes were retrieved during the early hours of August 3 and used for transplant. A 45-year-old man from Hyderabad who has cirrhosis of the liver and is in dire need of an organ transplant got a new lease of life by the liver donated at Global Hospital, Hyderabad. The kidney was donated to Global Hospital to save the life of a 43 –year old man who was on dialysis and waiting for an organ for more than a year. His eyes were donated to Swecha Gora Eye Bank in Vijayawada. Poet's daughter said, "My father had pledged his eyes several years ago. He was always positive and wanted to do something even after his death". (Credit: Times of India August 4, 2011)

3) Bangalore: *Woman gives new life to 5 after husband is declared brain-dead*: On Tuesday, 34 –year old Suparna's mind was with conflicting emotions. Back home in Kolkata, her near and dear ones were swaying to the beat of the drum during Durga Puja celebrations. But right before she lay her brain-dead husband. But there was no time to grieve. She has to take one of the most challenging decisions of her life: Should she donate his organs? Or Should she not...? Time was running out. The counsellor at the hospital had told her that organs should be harvested within six hours of a person being declared brain-dead. Shaking off her apprehensions and fighting off her tears, Suparna decided to give life to others instead. Nirmal Kumar's (name

changed) two kidneys, liver and eyes were successfully harvested and transplanted in five needy patients. Suparna's ordeal started when Nirmal, a businessman in his forties, suffered a massive brain haemorrhage last week. Suffering from hyper-sensitivity, he collapsed in his office and was wheeled into Columbia Asia Hospital. His condition was diagnosed as an intracranial haemorrhage-bleeding in the brain. After surgery, he was declared brain dead though his other organs were healthy. The hospital informed Suparna about organ donation during a counselling session that typically follows before the ventilators are taken off. A tearful Suparna, the mother of two school-going children, volunteered to donate Nirmal's organs. According to Dr. Chinnadurai R, consultant, critical care medicine at Columbia Asia Hospital, Nirmal Kumar was in a critical state when he was brought in due to continuous bleeding in the skull. "He could not pull through after the brain surgery and was brain-dead three days after. As part of our duties, we told his wife about organ donation and she agreed. It was indeed a bold step and she took the decision herself without informing her family as there could have been disagreements." Dr. Chinnadurai said. The family, originally from Kolkata, reside at Hebbal. Suparna's friends were quite surprised when she broke the news to them. "We could not believe what she was saying. Her husband was dying and she had decided to donate his organs. This doesn't come to everyone. She is a role model now and we plan to pledge our organs for donation." A friend said. (Credit: Bangalore Mirror October 27, 2012)

4) Bangalore: Paralytic man gives nine others a new lease of life: While watching a television programme on heart transplant about a month ago, Madhu R Shastry remarked to his father, "The brain is the only portion in my body which is not in working condition. The other organs are fine. You should donate all my organs." Madhu's father, Ramesha Krishnashastry, did not realise the gravity of his son's statement then, but it stayed in his mind. When 32 -year old Madhu was declared dead on Tuesday,

his family wasted no time deciding to donate his organs. Nine organs-kidneys, heart valves, corneas, and liver – were harvested and sent to the appropriate agencies. Madhu suffered from a congenital condition called brain arteriovenous malformation-an abnormal connection between arteries and veins in the brain. As a result, the right side was paralysed when he was ten years old, and he suffered from regular seizures. Due to his illness, Madu could not work and stayed at home doing distance education courses. He was constantly on medication, and his condition was monitored. His father, a retired Bosch employee, and mother, Gayathri, a music teacher, consulted several doctors, but Madhu's condition did not improve. On Sunday morning, he had an epileptic attack and collapsed. The family near Sanjayanager shifted him to a nearby hospital where doctors told them that their son's condition was critical. He had stopped responding to medication and was declared brain-dead. He was then transferred to Suguna Hospital in Rajajinagar. "The chances of his revival is nil", Dr. R Ravindra, medical director and chief of orthopaedics, Suguna Hospital, told Bangalore Mirror. "We informed his parents that he would only respond to life the support system. We were surprised when the father volunteered to his son's organs. The family had high levels of awareness about organ donation. Within three hours on Tuesday early morning, the organs were harvested and deposited. Since four heart valves were harvested, four heart patients awaiting for valve transplant were benefitted." While saddened by the loss, the family is also happy that even in death, Madhu gave life to nine others. "It's a mixed feeling," said Santosh Kumar, Madhu's brother-in-law. "He suffered for so long and now he is at peace while his organs are breathing life in someone else's body. We cannot get over what he told his father while watching that programme on heart transplantation. He had a big heart." (Credit: Bangalore Mirror August 14, 2014)

5) *I.A.S. Officer donates father's body to B.M.C.*: A senior I.A.S. officer of Karnataka, Dr. Shalini Rajneesh, has now donated the body of her father, who breathed his last on March 17. Late PP

Chhabra, also an I.A.S. officer, had pledged his body about five years ago in Faridabad. The organs of the 83- year- old retired I.A.S. who died of age-related complications had to be harvested within six hours from the time of his death. His body was given away to Bangalore Medical College and Research Institute (BMCRI), which will help students learn. The retired I.A.S. officer was a hero for his daughter in more than one and even in death set an example. "He was my role model and soon after we got his death certificate, my brothers and I decided to fulfil his last wish which I'm sure will inspire others." She said. Dr. Shalini Rajneesh promotes organ donation herself, urges people to pledge their organs, and has pledged her organs to Belgaum Medical College. "Most organs of person who has been declared brain-dead continue to function and can be useful to those who may need them, but because of social constraints, people don't feel comfortable donating them." She said, going on to add. "We did not hesitate as we think practically. My sense of morality told me that I should myself do what I've been asking others to do." According to a source from BMCRI, PP Chhabra's eyes have been given to Minto Eye Hospital, and the anatomy department of BMCRI is preserving the body. "Cadavers are important for medical colleges as they are used not only for medical research, but also for paramedical research. It can also be used by X-ray practitioners and to teach courses like physiotherapy. There is always a requirement for cadavers, as for a class of 250 under-graduation students, required 15-20 bodies," she said. (Credit: Bangalore Mirror March 23, 2017)

6) Bangalore: *Brain-dead man's organs donated:* A 43-year older man from Tumakuru, who met with an accident near D.L.F. Circle on April 24, has given a fresh lease of life to others with his family giving consent to donate his kidneys, liver and corneas. The man worked as a cashier at the bar near Jigani Circle and survived his wife, a 12-year-old son. On April 29, at about 9 PM, he was declared by the doctors as brain-dead at Narayana Health. "Due to head injuries he suffered during the bike-to-bike collision,

doctors diagnosed him with brain anoxia, wherein oxygen supply to the brain is cut off," said Srinivasan, the man's co-brother. His liver was transplanted to a 54 year -older man, while his left kidney had gone to a 38-year older man both at Narayan Healthcare. The right kidney went to a 42-year older adult at Apollo Hospitals. The corneas have been donated to Narayana Nethralaya. (Credit: Times of India May 5, 2019)

7) Bangalore: *Kin of two brain-dead patients donate organs*: Families of two people, who were declared brain-dead following accidents, decided to donate their organs, giving a new lease of life to over 13 people in 24 hours. In the first case, a 21-year-old labourer's liver and kidney were donated to Fortis Hospital Bannerghatta Road Bangalore and another kidney to I.N.U. Hospital, heart to Fortis Malar, Chennai and corneas to Netradhama Eye Hospital. In another case, a 30-year-old woman's liver and a kidney went to Fortis Hospital Bannerghatta Road Bangalore, Heart valve to Manipal Hospital, Corneas to Minto Eye Hospital, lungs to Fortis Malar, Chennai, another kidney to J.S.S. Hospital Mysore and small intestine and abdominal wall to Apollo Hospital, Chennai. (Credit: Times of India August 25, 2019)

8) New Delhi: *Four gets hope as brain-dead patient's kin donate organs*: At least four persons suffering from organ failure received a new lease of life on Friday when the family of a 43-year older woman, who was declared brain-dead at Apollo Hospital, consented to donate her organs. The woman's heart, liver and kidneys were retrieved when tests confirmed brain death. "A liver and kidneys were transplanted on two patients at Apollo while, as per the directions of National Organ and Tissue Transplant Organization (NOTTO), her heart was allocated to a hospital in Chennai", said Apollo Spokesperson. The 43-year old's second kidney was allocated to Human Care Medical Charitable Trust in Delhi. "It is difficult for any daughter to believe the fact that her mother is no longer with her. I was very close to her and will miss her every day. I wanted to keep her alive by any means. So when the doctors counselled us regarding donation

of her healthy organs, we agreed to it," the daughter of the deceased donor said. Poornima Shrivastava, the dead, was from Jhansi. Doctors said she was admitted to Apollo Hospital for a subarachnoid haemorrhage- bleeding in the space between the brain and the tissue covering the brain- on September 2. Despite treatment, her condition continued to deteriorate, and brain death was confirmed by apnoea tests recently. While living donors can only donate a portion of their liver or kidney, in case of brain death, multiple organs and tissues, including the heart, lungs, liver, kidneys, intestines, pancreas, eyes, heart valves, bone marrow, connective tissues, middle ear and blood vessels can be donated. (Credit: Times of India September 15, 2019)

Observance of special days to create awareness about health and organ donation:

Special campaigns are organised these days, such as bicycle and bike rallies, walkathons, marathons, workshops and seminars.

World Organ Donation Day:

August 13 every year is observed as Organ Donation Day. To motivate and encourage people to donate their organs and understand the value of organ donation in an individual's life. Who needs it because lakhs of people die every year waiting for an organ, and every 12 minutes, one more patient is added to the waiting list.

World Heart Day:

September 29 every year is celebrated as World Heart Day, Created by the Geneva-based World Heart Federation. It is a global campaign to inform people around the globe that 'cardiovascular disease' (CVD) refers to any disease of the heart, vascular disease of the brain, or infection of the blood vessel. According to the World Health Organization, it is the world's leading cause of death, claiming 17.9 million lives each year.

World Kidney Day:

2nd Thursday in March every year is celebrated as World Kidney Day. The International Society of Nephrology (ISN) and the International Federation of Kidney Foundations (IFKF) joint initiative. The event is a global campaign to raise awareness of the importance of our kidneys to our overall health. Many individuals and organisations worldwide celebrate this day by organising different activities to raise awareness of kidney disease.

World Liver day:

April 19 every year is observed as World Liver Day to spread awareness about the liver, the second-largest and the most complex organ in the body, except the brain. Liver diseases can be caused by hepatitis A, B, C, alcohol and drugs. Viral Hepatitis occurs due to consumption of contaminated food and water, unsafe sexual practices and drug abuse. If it is not treated on time, these can lead to Liver Cirrhosis and Liver Cancer. According to WHO, liver diseases are the 10th most common cause of death in India.

World Pancreatic Cancer Day:

November 21 every year is observed as World Pancreatic Cancer Day. People around the world unite to fight against the world's most challenging cancer. California based World Pancreatic Cancer Coalition, consisting of more than 80 organisations from over 30 countries and six continents. This body raises global awareness and inspired action, bringing greater attention, awareness, and better outcomes to this deadly disease.

World Lung Cancer Day:

August 1 every year is observed as World Lung Cancer Day. Lung cancer continues to be one of the most common cancers worldwide, claiming more lives yearly than breast, colon and prostate cancers combined. It is estimated that lung cancer accounts for nearly one in five cancer deaths globally.

It is heartening to know that organ donation registered three-fold growth in the last nine years. The efforts of the Government, hospitals and N.G.O.'s is showing success. India registered only 9000 liver, kidney and heart donations in 2009 against the figure of 3000 in 2018. In 2007-08, India collected 38000 corneas from dead persons, and the number rose to 68000 in 2018. But this number is insignificant as 10-15 lakhs individuals require corneal transplants in India.

One should pledge to donate the body and organs and encourage as many people as possible to do the same. We should cherish our priceless bodies and preserve life for the future by donating organs.

CHAPTER SEVEN

Philanthropic Activities and Health

The undertaking of philanthropic activities has a direct bearing on the health and happiness of an individual. One must involve in one, or the other acts of giving out of one's earning. The words philanthropy and charity are often used interchangeably, but there is a difference between these two concepts. The origin of the word Philanthropy comes from the Greek word, "Love of mankind". It is a private initiative for the public good which combines humanistic tradition with a social aspect. Charity comes from the French word Chrite which means "Providing for those in need; generosity and giving". The practice of charity involves giving money, goods, and labour by volunteering or time to the unfortunate, either directly or through a charitable trust.

Philanthropy attempts to address the root cause of the problem, while charity aims to relieve the pain of a particular social issue. An example is the difference between sending medicine and food to coronavirus disease patients, a charity. While educating the public in affected areas or supporting medical research in finding a cure for coronavirus disease is philanthropy. Charity tends to be an emotional, immediate response which mainly focuses on rescue and relief, whereas generosity is more strategic and built on rebuilding. Charity is giving. Philanthropy is acting and changing for a better world. Philanthropic acts support projects which will benefit all, such as libraries, museums and scientific research.

At the beginning of the 19th century providing free education to poor children was primarily among many philanthropists. Many people in the United States gave money to the causes in which they believe. Perhaps the most famous example of philanthropy came from Andrew Carnegie simply because of the scale of his giving. Carnegie's wealth helped build nearly 3000 libraries all over the world. Andrew Carnegie and John D. Rockefeller believed that responsibility to the less fortunate came with wealth. They established foundations to manage their wealth during and after their lifetimes.

Carnegie also endowed several universities and a charitable trust that runs nearly 100 years after his death in 1919. Another example is the Ford Foundation, established by the son of Ford Motor Company founder Henry Ford. The foundation focuses on strengthening democracy, improving economic opportunity, and advancing education.[1, 2]

Some people use philanthropy to gain recognition, prestige, power, name and fame. Some others think of charity as a way to gain the favour of the gods. Such things are normal because when wealth accumulates with any individual, he can use it how he wishes. We should be happy that at least he spends the wealth he created.

Volunteering is also generally considered an altruistic(selfless concern for other people's happiness and welfare)activity wherein an individual or group provides services to benefit another person, group or organisation. Volunteering has many positive benefits both for the volunteer as well as for the person or community served. It is also intended to make contacts for possible employment. Many volunteers are specifically trained in the areas they work in, such as medicine, education, or emergency rescue. Others serve on an as-needed basis, such as in response to a natural disaster.

Many heroes of philanthropists in India contributed their money and expertise to education, healthcare, creating jobs, and many more. Hurun Research Institute, in its India's Philanthropy

List 2018, stated that Indian philanthropy was at Rs 2310 crore, with an average donation per philanthropist being Rs 61 crore. They donated funds to develop education, social, rural development, livelihood creation, and healthcare. There were 21 self-made and 17 inherited entrepreneurs on the Hurun list. Mumbai houses the most philanthropists at 12, followed by Bengaluru (6) and Ahmedabad (4). The top 10 Indian philanthropists donated from October 1, 2017, to September 31, 2018. 1) Padma Bhushan awardee Shiv Nadar (Rs 770 crore) of the HCL, a multinational IT company. 2) Mukesh Ambani of Reliance Industries (Rs 437 crore), 3) Ajay Piramal and family (Rs 200 crore). 3) Azim Premji and family (Rs 113 crore) of Wipro IT Company. In 2013, he signed The Giving Pledge to donate at least half of his wealth, a campaign started by Bill Gates and Warren Buffett. So far, he has donated $ 21 billion to Azim Premji Foundation, an education-focused non-profit he founded in 2001. 4) Adi Godrej and family (Rs 96 crore) of the Godrej Group. His company supports the activities of the World Wildlife Fund in India. 5) Gautam Adani of the Adani Group (Rs 76 crore). 6) Yusuff Ali MA (Rs 70 crore) of Lulu Group International. 7) Savji Dholakia (Rs 40 crore) of the diamond exporting company 8) TATA Sons is owned by a philanthropic trust called TATA Philanthropic Allied Trusts, which contributes by tackling issues in health, education, and poverty. Similarly, every year several billionaires and millionaires donate their wealth for a public cause and upliftment of the poor worldwide.[3, 4]

Research Studies on Charitable Acts and Health:

Several research studies reveal that people who help others have healthier and happy lives. Doing well for others is good for us.

Dr. Stephen Post, Executive Director of the Unlimited Love Institute, a non-profit organisation, says: "There is a care-and-connection part of the brain. Brain studies show this profound state of joy and delight that comes from giving to others. It doesn't come from any dry action but acts like writing a cheque for a good cause and altruistic love".[5]

Stephen Post, a professor of preventive medicine at Stony Brook University, New York, reports that giving to others has been shown to increase health benefits in people with chronic illness, including HIV and multiple sclerosis. Stony Brook University has founded the Center for Medical Humanities, Compassionate Care, and Bioethics. The Center works with over 40 universities to better understand and teach compassionate care and its positive side effects.[6]

Stanford University has established a world-renowned centre aptly named the Center for Compassion and Altruism Research and Education (CCARE). Using a multidisciplinary approach, the Center's objective is to conduct research on compassion and altruism.

The University of California, Berkeley, the Greater Good Science Center conducts research in compassion and the six additional topics of gratitude, mindfulness, forgiveness, happiness, empathy, and altruism. The Center showcases its studies and many other outstanding research bodies under one roof using podcasts, articles, discussion forums, and events. Research by the Greater Good Science Center in Berkeley, California, supports the belief that being generous with others makes us happy. It is not only good for our health but also promotes social connection.

Further research suggests that charitable behaviour is the gift that keeps on giving back to the giver. "Helper's High" is a common phrase that originated in the late 1980s with Allan Luks, the Executive Director of the global Big Brothers and Big Sisters organisation. Luks was curious about the side effects of committing charitable acts and surveyed a sample of 3,000 adult volunteers. When the results came in, an astounding number of those surveyed – 95 per cent – experienced positive sensations or feelings after volunteering their services. Continuing his research in 2001, Luks and co-author, Peggy Payne wrote a book called The Healing Power of Doing Good –The Health and Spiritual

Benefits of Helping Others. The authors define Helper's High as a "euphoric feeling, followed by a long period of calm, experienced after performing a kind act." Their research also indicated that individuals who experience Helper's High routinely reported that they experienced fewer colds, increased joy and self-esteem, less stress, and even less physical pain.

In a 2006 study, Jorge Moll and colleagues at the National Institutes of Health found that when people give to charities, it activates brain regions associated with pleasure, social connection, and trust, creating a "warm glow" effect. Scientists also believe that altruistic behaviour releases endorphins in the brain, producing the "helper's high."

A 2007 study at Syracuse University noted that people with giving dispositions were 42 per cent more likely than non-givers to declare they were "very happy" and 25 per cent more likely to report they were "in excellent health." Happiness, it seems, instils us with a desire to make the world a better place. The inspiration to contribute to a more profound sense of belonging and community grows within.

A 2008 study by Harvard Business School professor Michael Norton and colleagues found that giving money to someone else lifted participants' happiness more than spending it on themselves (despite participants' prediction that spending on themselves would make them happier). Happiness expert Sonja Lyubomirsky, a professor of psychology at the University of California, Riverside, saw similar results when she asked people to perform five acts of kindness each week for six weeks.

A wide range of research has linked different forms of generosity to better health, even among the sick and elderly. A 1999 study led by Doug Oman of the University of California, Berkeley, found that older people who volunteered for two or more organisations were 44 per cent less likely to die over five years than non-volunteers, even after controlling for their age, exercise habits, general health, and adverse health habits like smoking.

Stephanie Brown of the University of Michigan saw similar results in a 2003 study on elderly couples. She and her colleagues found that those who provided practical help to friends, relatives, or neighbours, or gave emotional support to their spouses, had a lower risk of dying over five years than those who didn't. Interestingly, receiving help wasn't linked to reduced death risk.

Researchers suggest that giving may improve physical health and longevity because it helps decrease stress, which is associated with various health problems. In a 2006 study by Rachel Pierri of Johns Hopkins University and Kathleen Lawler of the University of Tennessee, people who provided social support to others had lower blood pressure than participants who didn't, suggesting a direct physiological benefit to those who give of themselves.

A study by James Fowler of the University of California, San Diego, and Nicholas Christakis of Harvard, published in the Proceedings of the National Academy of Science, shows that when one person behaves generously, it inspires observers to act well later, toward different people. The researchers found that altruism could spread by three degrees—from person to person. "As a result," they write, "each person in a network can influence dozens or even hundreds of people, some of whom he or she does not know and has not met."

Giving donations has also been linked to oxytocin, a hormone (also released during sex and breastfeeding) that induces feelings of warmth, euphoria, and connection to others. In laboratory studies, Paul Zak, the director of the Center for Neuroeconomics Studies at Claremont Graduate University, has found that a dose of oxytocin will cause people to give more generously and feel more empathy towards others "symptoms" lasting up to two hours. And those people on an "oxytocin high" can potentially jumpstart a "virtuous circle, where one person's generous behavior triggers another's," says Zak. [7, 8]

The World Giving Index, run by Charities Aid Foundation (CAF) in the United Kingdom, has a mission "to motivate society to give ever more effectively, helping to transform lives and communities around the world." Each year, this foundation studies 135 countries. It ranks them based on their citizens' charitable behaviours and actions in the last 30 days, specifically focusing on monetary donations, volunteering time, and helping a stranger. In addition, the World Giving Index survey also showed that happiness had more influence than wealth on how much money was given away. This finding connects well with other research, which shows us that the happier you are, the more optimistic you are about yourself, your actions, and those around you. Happiness instils us with a desire to make the world a better place. The inspiration to contribute to a more profound sense of belonging and community grows within.

Some communities subscribe to cultivating collective happiness as a standard for living. The country of Bhutan has become known worldwide for creating the Gross National Happiness Index (GNH). The GNH index uses nine domains (psychological well-being, time use, community vitality, cultural diversity, ecological resilience, living standards, health, education, and good governance) to provide a breakdown of happiness in alignment with Bhutanese culture. The GNH Index sees the pursuit of happiness as a community or collective happiness, although it is also experienced individually. Jigme Thinley, the first elected Prime Minister of Bhutan, said about the concept of happiness and community "We know that true abiding happiness cannot exist while others suffer, and comes only from serving others, living in harmony with nature, and realising our innate wisdom and the true and brilliant nature of our own minds."

Religious roots of Charity:

Throughout history, the most violent wars have been fought over religion. Even today, the world is divided by religious faiths; however, altruism is one aspect practised in all the significant beliefs.

All religions teach their followers from a very young age to give to the poor through material wealth and volunteering. These religious faiths have long-established schools, hospitals and social service organisations for the benefit of the public at large.

There is another class of non-believers of any deities-Atheists (nearly one billion), which is the fastest-growing group in the world. This group is also humanists undertaking many activities of brotherhood and compassion for the less privileged and poor. The top atheist's countries where the atheist population ranges between 52 to 77 per cent are Estonia, Czech Republic, Japan, Denmark, Sweden, Vietnam, Macau, Hong Kong, France and Norway. The world's faithful account for 83 per cent, while atheists constitute about 17 per cent of the global population. The fundamental belief to assist the poor practised in all major religions indicates that we are not so different from each other no matter what faith we practice. Another thing is the rich and poor class exist for ages. The cycle of the poor becoming rich and vice versa has lived for generations.

The late American author and founder of The Human Kindness Foundation, Bo Lozoff, wrote: "In the midst of global crises such as pollution, wars and famine, kindness may too easily be dismissed as a soft issue or a luxury to be addressed after more urgent problems are solved. But kindness is in the greatest of need in all those areas. Kindness toward the environment, toward other nations, and toward the needs of people suffering. Simple kindness may be the most vital key to the riddle of how human beings can live with each other and care properly for this planet we all share."

Generosity does not depend on the monetary value but more on the intention to help and serve. It could be anyone say time, talent and money or combining all the three. The fundamental belief to assist the poor practised in all major religions gives hope that we are not so different from each other no matter what faith we practice. All organised religions have traditionally played a significant role in charitable works such as establishing schools, hospitals and social service organisations.

Christianity

One of the most important texts of Christianity, the Sermon on the Mount, says if you help the needy, you comfort the suffering ones - you do good not only for them but for Jesus Christ, as well. Followers must live wisely and cheerfully rather than for praise and admiration from others. Giving should be for an act of glory of God and the good of His people. Christians believe money and possessions are irrelevant as something beyond this world is better, and they put their faith to provide in God. Many Christians support their churches and clergy with monetary contributions of one kind or another. Frequently, this is called tithing. Jesus would say, "Life is God's gift to us. How we live is our gift to God." Regardless of their income level and circumstances, everyone is encouraged to give something regularly and consider the gift and its amount thoughtfully and prayerfully. We are also encouraged to share our first fruits, as opposed to what is left over. In this way, we make the needs of God's church, and its ministry, a priority in our life. Tithing is a commandment accepted by various churches in the Latter Day Saint movement. Adherents make generous tithe donations, usually ten per cent of their income, to their church.

Islam

In Islam, it is mandatory to provide a charitable contribution, as it is the right of the poor to find relief from the rich and is considered a tax or obligatory alms. Typically charity is given around the month of Ramadan but can be made at any time, to anyone. Giving, also called sadaqah, can take various forms: money, clothing, knowledge and shelter. It is compulsory for Muslims who can afford to give in different forms of giving. The one that is best known is zakat or almsgiving—one of the Five Pillars of Islam. It is usually defined as a mandatory way of redistributing wealth. In the days of Islamic empires, it was very much institutionalised, like a tax system, where citizens were expected to give a percentage of their income to satisfy the community's needs. In the modern world, we see charity as a much more personal act, but it was much more a community duty in the ancient Islamic world. When Prophet Mohammed was asked, "What if a person has nothing?" The Prophet replied, "He should work with his own hands for his benefit and then give something out of such earnings in charity." Each person, every mosque, all families, regardless of age and language, donate 2.5% of their income yearly because, in the words of the Quran, to save one life is to protect the entire human race.

Buddhism

More than two and a half thousand years ago, Gautama Buddha recommended charity as one of the paths to enlightenment. Charity involves material giving, giving of fearlessness and giving of dharma. Material giving consists of food to the hungry, shelter to the homeless and money to the poor. Sharing Buddhist teachings with others is dharma. The act of giving voluntarily in Buddhism is motivated by a recognition that all beings exist in interdependence. The interdependence of all things, combined with an awareness of the helplessness of those less fortunate, inspires compassion. Practising selflessness in this way increases one's merit and is also an antidote to greed or grasping possessions or other resources. Giving is an expression of the natural qualities of kindness and compassion. Recognition of the interdependence of life also means taking care of the environment by keeping it pure and unspoiled and attending to animals and spirits in some traditions by offering prayers, rituals, ceremonies, or other acts dedicated to the well-being of all life. Traditionally, Buddhists emphasise giving alms, food, medicine, and clothing to monks and monasteries in exchange for teachings and merit. This relationship is seen as a sacred mutual dependence. The merit (Punya) is shared on both sides for the benefit of all. Teachings about karma (deeds) explain that our past actions affect us positively or negatively and that our present actions will affect us in the future. Buddhism uses an agricultural metaphor to explain how sowing good or bad seeds will result in good or bad fruit.

Hinduism

All Hindu scriptures state that the three characteristics of a good person are damah (self-restraint), daya (compassion or love for all life) and daana (charity). Karmayoga is the primary path of salvation (Mukti). It prescribes not only donating wealth but also service and sacrifice. Charity is more than just giving; it involves sharing resources with others, wealth, food, or other things. Daana has been defined in traditional texts as any action of surrendering the ownership of what one considered or identified as one's own and investing the same in a recipient without expecting anything in return. Hinduism lay a great emphasis on the act of giving away part of your income. The Upanishads, a text containing the philosophical concepts of Hinduism, talks about daana (giving to an individual, in distress or need, as an act of virtue). As per the Upanishads, Daana can also take philanthropic public projects that empower and help many. Historical records indicate that daana is an ancient practice in Indian traditions, tracing back to Vedic rites. The Rig Veda, one of the four sacred texts in Hinduism, contains the earliest discussion of daana. The Rig Veda relates it to Satya (truth) and the guilt of not giving to those in need.

The choultries in India are one expression of Hindu charity. The choultries are shelters, or rest houses, for travellers and the poor, with much serving water and free food. These are usually built along the roads that connect to major Hindu temple sites. All Hindu temples serve as charitable institutions. They collect donations (daana) from devotees, which are used to feed people in distress and fund public projects. Swami Dayanand Saraswati, the founder of the Arya Samaj Movement, recommended giving away one-hundredth of one's income to charity. In Hinduism, some rituals occur around main festivals, and no practice is considered complete without daana.

Judaism

In Judaism, tzedakah (charity) is a fundamental part of the Jewish way of life. It is a form of social justice provided by the donor. A percentage of income is given to charity. However, it is about giving money and showing compassion and empathy along with the donation. Traditional Jewish homes commonly have a pushke, a box for collecting coins for the poor. Orthodox Jews give at least ten per cent of their net income to charity. The obligation to perform tzedakah can be fulfilled by giving money to the poor, health care institutions, synagogues, or educational institutions.

Sikhism:

It is one of the youngest world religions, founded by Guru Nanak in the early sixteenth century. Guru Nanak has an interesting perspective for salvation: Pilgrimage, penance, compassion, and charitable giving. Guru Nanak provides Sikhs with a new ethical framework in which people who are fit to work are required to earn a living through honest means while sharing the fruits of their earnings with sections of society that are the neediest. This theology can be summed up in his famous pronouncement recorded in the Guru Granth Sahib, the Sikh scripture: 'Only they are on the True Path who eat what they earn through earnest work and help support the disenfranchised'. One institution that comes out of this ethical framework is the langar (free community kitchen). The Darbar Sahib—also known as the Golden Temple—in Amritsar, Panjab, serves food daily to 100,000 people, regardless of their status or religious affiliation. As a consequence, it is said, no one in Amritsar has slept hungry in the last four centuries. Similarly, wherever Gurudwara is in the world, there is a langer attached to provide food. [9,10,11,12]

My social service activities:

1. Rural Development Officer: While serving at Syndicate Bank, Koppal, I took the initiative to ensure farmers get credit and the latest technologies as per the policy of Syndicate Bank at that time. In this regard, I volunteered my time beyond office hours and even on holidays. Farmers were interested in adopting new crops, varieties, cultivation practices, value addition, and marketing. I initiated several extension activities to expose them

to new technologies and successful farmers in Karnataka and neighbouring states. For instance: Mango- Panem in Andhra Pradesh to get high yielding good quality planting material; Grapes- Tasgaon in Maharashtra; Plantation crops; Kasaragod in Kerala. I coordinated and led the farmer group to these places. I even put leave and shared the expenses with farmers, including deposit customers and farm loan clients. The farmers were so impressed and motivated by these trips that many farmers established new mango and coconut orchards on scientific lines. Of course, the situation is entirely different now after four decades as water scarcity compelled the farmers to go in for still high-value crops like pomegranate and hybrid seed production in cotton, field crops, flowers and vegetables. But the excellent relationship I built with these farmers is that we still exchange greetings on festivals and other occasions as good human beings and friends beyond bank and customer relationships.

2. Mumbai: When I was working in Mumbai, I was closely associated with Havyaka Welfare Trust, a charitable trust established in 1964, involved in social-cultural activities with nearly one thousand members. The trust maintained two medical centres and a hostel for students. Medical centres provided service to the public at a concessional rate. The trust regularly organised health check-up camps. The trust also brought out a bilingual monthly Kannada and English journal containing general interest news and articles. I was the honorary chief editor of this journal for eight years while working in Mumbai (1996 to 2004). I was also actively involved in fundraising events of the trust. I also brought out one directory containing details of trust's members, which enabled better communication.

3. Ramakrishna Math and Ramakrishna Mission, Khar, Mumbai: is a branch of its Head Quarter at Belur, Howrah. The institution forms the core of a worldwide spiritual movement. It aims to harmonise religions, a harmony of the East and the West, harmony of the ancient and the modern, spiritual fulfilment,

all-round development of human faculties, social equality, and peace for all humanity, without any distinctions of creed, caste, race or nationality. It is one of the oldest centres of the Ramakrishna Order, established in 1923. It has provided solace to hundreds of individuals who seek inner peace beyond the hustle of daily life, particularly in a city like Mumbai. It also offers dedicated service to the needy in and around Mumbai – with the attitude of 'Service to man is worship of God'.

The Math centre activities comprise daily worship and bhajans, celebrations of different Hindu festivals, birthdays of Sri Ramakrishna, Holy Mother Sri Sharada Devi, Sri Swami Vivekananda, and other religious personages conducting religious classes and spiritual retreats. Mission activities include establishing a hospital, a library in Mumbai and a Rural Development Centre at Sakwar, situated on the Mumbai-Ahmedabad Highway about 82 km from Mumbai in Vasai Taluka of Palghar District.

The centre was established in 1972 to serve people residing in about 500 backward villages nearby. People lacked easy access to medical services, education and even occupation to earn any income. The monks and volunteers, including doctors, conduct medical camps every Sunday in Sakwar centre. It also has a small agriculture demonstration farm.

Volunteer doctors and volunteers carry medical services at the centre. The facilities include X-Ray, automated pathology lab, nursing station and consulting rooms. The patients are given free medicines, vitamins, proteins etc. and nutritious lunches. Patients requiring hospitalisations are admitted to the Mission hospital in Mumbai or admitted to nearby hospitals.

I was associated with rural development activities at Sakwar when working in Mumbai. Frequently on Sundays, I travelled to Sakwar along with monk in charge and doctors to provide technical expertise for its agriculture farm and vocational training centre. Vocational training centre offered courses in tailoring, carpentry, electric wiremen, motor vehicles mechanic, motor driver cum mechanic, welding (gas & electrical), a community health worker. Besides, the students are also imparted spiritual training. Apart from the regular training, students also participate in cultural events and work on the campus in the dairy farm, agriculture field, which provides extensive practical experience and moulded their personality. Besides this, the students are also imparted spiritual training.

I am proud to say that I prepared a project seeking grants from an organisation with corporate social responsibility. The project was designed and monitored. I ensured the full release of the funds and the successful completion of the project. I helped them to raise orchards with improved varieties of fruits. As per my suggestion, a 'Panchavati' is also set up wherein five sacred trees are planted as per the Vedic scripture. Panchavati should have five trees planted in the following direction. Aswath or Bodhi or Peepal tree- *Ficus religiosa on the* East; Aonla or Indian gooseberry *-Emblica officinalis* on the South; Bael-*Aegle marmelos* on the North; Banyan-*Ficus benghalensis* on the West; Ashoka *-Saraca indica* on the South East. These trees have not only tremendous pollution-fighting capacity but also maintain ecological balance. Each part of these trees is helpful to human beings and animals as they produce food, fodder, timber and medicines for many ailments. I also remember the help rendered by Mr Gulabrao Patil, who then worked with NGO-BAIF in a bio-diversity conservation project at Ghansoli in Thane district.

4. Community service in my apartment: I took the keen initiative to in-situ community composting from green waste as a part of decentralised solid waste management in Bengaluru. I live in a 192 unit apartment wherein 100 kg green waste is available for composting on an average daily. For any sustainable solid waste management project, waste segregation at the source is a prerequisite. Hence, I took the lead to create awareness and educate residents by putting up a series of circulars in the notice

boards from time to time with appropriate pictorial charts for segregation into different categories at home. The committed team members had several meetings to discuss the issue and how to involve residents. I was a core team member responsible for installing an aerobic wet waste digester in my complex.

5. School for the hearing and speech impaired children, Sirsi: I started donating a fixed sum every month since I retired from bank service in 2007, and I like to continue till my last breath. The school was established in my native place in 1981, which provides education from 1ˢᵗto 10ᵗʰstandard admitting both boys and girls. The money goes directly from my pension crediting account to the school account, similar to any recurring deposit. I selected this institution because the school admits children from all castes, and I feel the students are God's children. During my visit to my native place, I visit the school and get the satisfaction that my donation is used for a good cause. Looking at my gesture, one of my younger brothers is also donating every year. Further, we have not allowed the school to publicise our kind gesture.

After retirement, I also sponsored a room in the hospital constructed by a charitable trust in my native place. Besides this, my contribution has gone to many educational institutions but under an anonymous donor list. I feel such good deeds are leading me to a confident, peaceful, and stress-free life.

The pandemic Covid-19 had opened the door for philanthropic activities for all to help the distressed in India. Millions of migrant guest workers from north India were experiencing a lack of food and transport facilities to return to native places when the nationwide lockdown was declared in 2020. At the same time, many entrepreneurs arranged kits containing food grains and groceries. Kind people opened many makeshift kitchens to provide thousands of hot meals every day. As per their capacity, donors supplied in all forms, say cash, kind and voluntary service. Some even offered their vehicles for transport. This act of generosity towards the poor was a great charity towards fellow human beings. Some people even hired chartered flights to send the guest migrant workers home from one state to another during the lockdown.

The Covid -19 pandemic taught a lesson to everybody that death is a lonely one. Loved ones, family or friends do not want to get a glimpse of the departed, fearing infection though the body is wrapped in three-layer protective material. However, it is reported that Mercy Angels, a wing of NGO Mercy Mission, a six-member team of volunteers including a doctor, is ensuring those who died of the virus in Bengaluru get a dignified funeral. Cremation or burial also does not cost the bereaved families. They wait for the call from the hospital mortuary and transport the corpse to a funeral or burial place. Such great noble acts are honest service to humanity.

Another act of heart touching service to the community as appeared in the press is appended here.

Cleanliness service by an advocate for sanitising places of worship: Visakhapatnam: With questions around hygiene assuming significance amid the pandemic, practising advocate, mountaineer and state National Service Scheme (NSS) awardee MGM Khan has taken upon himself the task of single-handedly sanitising places of worship of different religions.

Through his actions, the 27-year-old hopes that residents and authorities at places of worship realise the importance of cleanliness as a safeguard against the coronavirus.

An exercise started as a sanitising service in mosques during Ramzan on May 10, 2020, soon extended to temples, churches and Gurudwaras in Vizag city. So far, Khan has sanitised 22 mosques, 11 temples, 8 churches and a Gurudwara using around 1500 litres of sanitising spray (a solution of sodium hypochlorite, ammonium chloride and camphor). His target is to utilise one lakh litre of non-alcoholic sanitising solution and include Anganwadi (child care centres) in clean-up drives in future.

For temples, Khan went a step forward and mixed a few drops of holy Ganges water from the upper reaches of Gangotri, which he had collected in January while on a mountaineering and skiing course at Uttarakashi."Initially, some people of my community asked why I am bothered about cleaning churches and temples. The Quran Hadees directs us to serve humanity. I felt it is my responsibility to extend social service for humanity because Covid-19 can attack followers of any religion and hence all these places need cleansing. Also, I am inspired by Ratan Tata's words who said the motto of 2020 is not about earning but about living and I believe prevention is always better than cure," said Khan, who is also a yoga teacher.

Many places of worship have offered to pay him for his service, but Khan has refused and accepted Rs2 as a symbolic gesture. He has spent nearly Rs 50000 so far and carries on his back a 20- litre spraying machine while setting out for work.

"As more people came to know, I recently got offers from Christian minority body to sanitise 50 churches and I also intend to offer my service to Jain temple authorities. But all places of worship should maintain a sanitising machine and get the premises and interiors sanitised every week," said Khan. The advocate, who has an MSc yoga degree from Chennai, an MA psychology degree from Andhra University (AU) and an LLB from AU Law College, is currently pursuing an LLM from NBM Law College, thanked his family for supporting his endeavours. (Credit: Times of India, June 11, 2020).

CHAPTER EIGHT

Experience with Nature Cure

One week Course at Nature Cure Centre, Urulikanchan, Pune:

At the instance of Mahatma Gandhiji, the nature cure centre was established. When Gandhiji was in South Africa, he suffered from chronic stomachache, which was cured through naturopathy. He was also motivated by reading a book, "Return to Nature", written by Adolf Just (1859-1936), a German naturopath. He was a strong advocate of natural remedies utilising natural food, clean water, fresh air, earthen clay, and good time spent in greenery. Gandhiji had an idea to set up one naturopathy centre in India to promote its concept among the common people. In this background, this centre was established in 1946 at Urulikanchan, near Pune.

The main aim of the nature cure treatment centre is to educate the people and create awareness about health and hygiene. In Naturopathy, it is emphasised on educating a person about the right way of living and management of health problems in simple ways. People experience the effect of living following the laws of Nature. Naturopathy believes that all diseases are equal, but our lifestyle leads to different diseases. Purification of mind and body is vital to remove the root cause of diseases. By following the laws of Nature, elimination of toxins from the body is possible, which helps to improve vitality and immunity. Natural food such as fruits and vegetables in juices –salad- sprouts-boiled vegetables-baked potatoes-sweet potatoes are used as medicines.

All-natural foodstuffs are rich in natural water, vitamins, minerals and roughage. It helps eliminate toxins through the increased quantity of urine, proper bowel movements through regulation of breath & improved metabolism. Natural food balances metabolism, blood sugar, blood urea, uric acid, cholesterol, lipids etc. which is achieved without drugs. The treatment is based on five natural elements, i.e. Ether(*Aakash*), Sunlight *(Tej)*, Air *(Vayu)*, Water *(Jal)* and Earth *(Prithvi)*.

Nature cure practices are the best way to keep the diseases away from our bodies, but it does not always happen. I quote here that I suffered over a decade from Irritable Bowel Syndrome (IBS), which ultimately proved that it is not a disease. But by that time, it had made room for another disease to pile in my body. While IBS is related to mind pile relates to part of the body. Whenever I approached doctors complaining about IBS, they told me that nothing happens even if I do not pass poop for two to three days. The body will not keep the digested food for a long time. But my mind was the culprit. My mind was saying that the bowel should be out entirely before going to the office. Hence, I spent a lot of time in the toilet emptying the bowels by straining, which led to piles.

At a later stage, a protruded rectum was causing much embarrassment. The pile is such an awkward disease neither we can express openly nor stop doing daily routine work. When I was working in Mumbai, one of my colleagues and I visited Bombay Hospital sometime in 1986 just for a check-up. But the doctor said, "Nothing to worry. Give half an hour I will cure the disease conducting painless cryosurgery, right now". We were delighted and instantly agreed. Before knowing what cryosurgery was, the doctor finished the operation, collected INR 900 from each, and sent us out. Later, we realised the extreme cold, even up to minus 40 degrees C produced by liquid nitrogen, and destroys abnormal tissues or haemorrhoids, swollen blood vessels in the anal canal. However, in 1996 I had to go for removal of the protruded rectum through surgery. Surgeon Dr. Thomas cautioned me. While discharging, "Mr.Hegde, if you sit in the toilet for more than five minutes now onwards, we have to operate again. Be careful". Thank God, since then pile has not relapsed.

In 1999, when my best friend, the Managing Trustee for a Nature Cure Centre, Urulikanchan near Pune, suggested undergoing one week course, I heeded his advice. I stayed here for a week just for relaxation and rejuvenation when working in Mumbai. However, I had no ailment requiring any treatment—The published article on my experience in the nature cure centre, Urulikanchan, in 2000.

Uruli Kanchan-Pune Ashram shows the way back to Mother Nature: Since I was longing to be alone entirely away from routine work of attending home, office, travel, telephones and meetings etc. and I thank my friend who suggested me a proper place Uruli Kanchan Nature Cure Ashram, Pune. I reached Pune on Sunday evening to join Ashram schedule from Monday.

The beginning of this Ashram is exciting to know. Father of Nation Mahatma Gandhi, a firm believer in the philosophy of nature cure, wanted naturopathy to benefit the rural poor. He established this Ashram (Trust) in 1946. He entrusted the execution responsibility to his trusted disciples, the two of young inspired bachelors, social reformer Late Dr. Manibhai Desai and spiritual leader Balkoba Bhave, the brother of Vinoba Bhave, the crusader of Bhoodaan Movement in India. Gandhiji stayed in this Ashram during 22-30 March 1946. Since then, Ashram has been promoting the science of curing diseases without any drugs through treatment tools like food, fasting, steam-baths, sun-baths, mud-baths and massage, water therapy, walks, herbs, and health habits, prayers, yoga, meditation and acupressure etc. It has made remarkable progress in promoting nature cure, community health, hygiene and sanitation and is professionally managed by a dedicated team of Naturopaths.

Urulikanchan is a small town situated on National Highway No.9 at 30 km from Pune on Sholapur road. The Ashram lies amidst serene and scenic natural greenery. One can breathe fresh air, get farm-fresh fruits and vegetables, plenty of cow milk and tender coconut water. One can hear the musical chirping of birds throughout the day. Discipline, austerity, humanism, hygiene and self-help are the hallmarks of this Ashram which sprawls over 25 acres.

The well-planned Nature Cure Institute is laid out on 10 acres. Another 15 acres was added to grow Mother Nature's bounty crops of food, flower, fruits, medicinal plants, and forests. The green environment is bringing soothing effects human mind and body. One can see extensively grown Tulsi or holy basil (*Ocimum tenuiflorum*) over an area of more than one acre, so also other crops like papaya and lemongrass.

On the day of the visit on December 25, 1999, there were 111 patients (now the capacity is 220 in 2021) on the roster. Out of which 39 male and female 72 female, of all age groups ranging from 8 to 80 who came from all corners of India and abroad, seeking relief from mild to chronic ailments. However, 3 to 6 months advance booking is required. There are different buildings like a hospital, library, community kitchen, dining hall, prayer cum yoga hall, office, well laid out garden. Walkers count round after rounds both morning and evening in the park. Four rounds make one kilometre. The library has over 10,000 books collected over 50 years and a sale counter where one could get any book on food, nutrition and naturopathy in different Indian languages and English. The library also subscribes to periodicals and journals on naturopathy from the world over.

There are separate treatment wards for ladies and gents. These wards have several rooms to administer different treatments like hydrotherapy anima, hip bath, tub bath, full-body sauna steam bath, wet abdominal cold-hot water pack, hot water feet bath, spinal bath sun-bath and abdominal or local wet clay mud pack etc. Massaging by well-trained male massagers will be done either in the rooms or on the terrace for males under the sun and female massagers for ladies in their respective rooms. One could see three big boilers working for 6 hours a day to provide the required hot water and steam for the whole body. Everything goes as per the prescription of the dedicated naturopaths, all of whom stay in the Ashram only.

The Ashram doctors say, "It is pity that mostly who come here are those who have failed with other types of medicines say allopath, homeopathy or Ayurveda. They come not with faith and confidence but due to compulsion as a last resort for cure. It should not be the case. People should realise the benefit of following principles of naturopathy as a preventive measure for diseases and also for their cure".

Naturopathy adopts a holistic approach by combining fasting, changing food habits, blending yoga, prayer, exercise, meditation, etc. Live natural positive food like sprouts, vegetables, fruits and milk are believed to work as medicine for purification of body and mind. Fasting on water, fruit juices, tender coconut water, yoga and other treatments help in the elimination of toxic matter from the body.

Patients with chronic functional and psycho-somatic diseases like arthritis, asthma, digestive disorders, hypertension, depression and heart diseases, diabetes, skin diseases like eczema and psoriasis, obesity, spondylitis and various gynaecological disorders are also very well managed by simple procedures and diet control.

My daily routine in the Ashram from 5 AM to 9 PM were: Brisk walk, prayer and exercise under the guidance of yoga teacher, whole-body massage from toe to head by expert massager Sun-bath and abdominal wet mud pack, sauna steam bath and full body tub bath, attending discourse on yoga, meditation, naturopathy and holistic health Community prayer, self-study & meditation etc.

Lunch and dinner comprised of pure vegetarian wholesome food, rotis (chapati or phulka) made out of wheat or jowar (Sorghum a millet) flour, two vegetables, green salad and a bowl of kichdi (a dish made out of rice and green gram) which were devoid of salt. Food used to be served under the strict supervision of the community kitchen supervisor. Passion foods such as onion, garlic, meat, fish and eggs and beverages like tea, coffee or cola etc., are strictly taboo in the Ashram. Fruit juices, curd and only herbal tea (Kada) are served depending on the patient's need. Kada with the recipe of water, jaggery, tulsi leaves, ginger and lemongrass, which makes a perfect grandma medicine.

There are different types of accommodation to suit the pockets of all classes (general ward, single/double rooms and cottages). Ashram has also given employment to local people who are very courteous. Both ladies and gents work as cooks, room attendants, massagers, laundrymen and laundry women, attendants to administer different therapies from dawn to dusk. I felt relaxed and returned with a desire to go once again for a more extended period.

Ashram attracts hundreds of visitors daily from all over India and abroad. It has turned into an Institute of Excellence. It spreads the message that Mother Nature cures diseases and takes care of our ailments, provided we have faith and strong will to follow her principles. Vedic scriptures also prescribe that all five sensory organs (eye, ear, tongue, nose and skin) and five work organs (mouth, hands, legs, rectum and urethra) should function properly to be healthy. If one of these ten organs malfunctions, we face health issues. Humans have five vital organs that are essential for survival. These are the brain, heart, kidneys, liver and lungs. Fascinating facts about our body are: The human body contains nearly 100 trillion cells; there are at least ten times as many bacteria in the human body as cells; the average adult takes over 20,000 breaths a day; each day, the kidneys process about 200 quarts (50 gallons) of blood to filter out about 2 quarts of waste and water; adults excrete about a quart and a half (1.42 litres) of urine each day; the human brain contains about 100 billion nerve cells; water makes up more than 50 per cent of the average adult's body weight.

Nature Cure Beliefs: More dishes, more diseases; More medicines, more miseries; More comforts more complaints; One should eat what one requires; Food should become the medicine; Be health conscious not disease conscious; More relief more grief; More drugs more doubts; More nourishment more punishment; Good health is the foundation of life; Common sense and will power health; Beware of three white poisons: sugar, salt and *maida* (finely milled wheat flour without any bran, refined, and bleached, it closely resembles cake flour).

Traditional naturopaths deal exclusively with changes in diet and lifestyle and do not generally recommend vaccines and antibiotics. In India, naturopathy is overseen by the Ministry of Ayurveda, Yoga and Naturopathy, Unani, Siddha and Homoeopathy (AYUSH).[1] There is a 5½-year "Bachelor of Naturopathy and Yogic Sciences" (BNYS) degree that twelve colleges in India offer. The National Institute of Naturopathy in Pune operates under AYUSH, established on December 22, 1986. It facilitates standardisation and propagation of the existing knowledge and its application through research in naturopathy throughout India. It is learnt that now the Nature Cure Centre, Urulikanchan is also a documentation centre on naturopathy.

The use of complementary and alternative medicine (CAM) is increasing rapidly, which includes naturopathy also. The World Health Organization (WHO) classifies 65–80% of the world's health care services as 'traditional medicine'. Therefore, from the viewpoint of the population ratio, more people use CAM than modern western medicine. However, scientific evidence for most CAM is still sparse. However, CAM has become so popular among 'consumers' due to reasons like: Non-invasive with few side effects, helps to improve quality of life, helps one to maintain one's health, modern Western medicine does not fully correspond to the patients' demands, the trend towards a more holistic medical approach, ballooning medical expenses etc. For example, the current status of CAM in Japan is unique and noteworthy since highly advanced modern Western medicine coexists with traditional medicine.[2]

However, for every ailment, nature cure is not the answer. Thanks to innovations in modern medical sciences. In case of degeneration of body organs, surgeries, transplants, and implants are doing wonders for the longevity of human beings.

CHAPTER NINE

A Student of Vipassana Meditation

In 2001 when I was working in Mumbai, I visited the Kalina campus of the Mumbai University to enquire about a diploma course in Yoga for my wife since she had evinced interest. While looking in the notice board, I also noticed "One year part time diploma course in Buddhism and Vipassana". Suddenly I recollected my memory while studying history in high school, incidents about King Ashoka, the war of Kalinga, and later who followed non-violence when he came across with Buddha's teachings the Dhamma(Dharma). Interestingly, though Ashoks's period was about 250 years after the Buddha's passing away (nirvana) but Ashoka, who was obsessed with power, became Dhamma Ashoka. He inspired his citizens to walk on this path and spread the message to neighbouring countries. Somehow my desire kindled to undergo this course. The course was offered every Saturday from 3:00 to 5:30 PM. During next week I paid the fees and registered for the course. The course syllabus comprised of an introduction to Pali language, the definition of Tipitaka(the Buddhist sacred scriptures or Pali canon), advantages of learning Pali, opening to life and teachings of Buddha, four Noble Truths(First-suffering; Second-origin of suffering; Third-cessation of suffering; Fourth-eightfold path to the cessation of suffering), historical places connected with the life of Buddha and also Vipassana theory and practice. Attending a 10-Day Vipassana meditation course at Dhammagiri, Vipassana International

Academy, Igatpuri near Nashik was also a part of the course.[1]

What is Vipassana?

The technique of Vipassana is a simple, practical way to achieve real peace of mind and to lead a happy, helpful life. Vipassana means "to see things as they really are". It is a logical process of mental purification through self-observation. From time to time, we all experience agitation, frustration and disharmony. When we suffer, we do not keep our misery limited to ourselves; instead, we distribute it to others. Indeed, this is not a proper way to live. We all want to live peacefully within ourselves and with those around us. After all, human beings are social beings: we have to live and interact with others. How, then, can we live peacefully? How, then, can we remain harmonious ourselves and maintain peace and harmony around us? Vipassana enables us to experience peace and harmony by purifying the mind, freeing it from suffering and the deep-seated causes of suffering. Step by step, the practice leads to the highest spiritual goal of total liberation from all mental defilements.

Vipassana, a Pali word, means to see things as they are. The meditation technique was rediscovered by Gautama, the Buddha (560-480 B.C.) in India to ease universal suffering to cope with the various conflicts we face in our day-to-day life.

Meditation Procedure:

We have to sit down cross-legged, closing our eyes. Then, we have to focus our attention around our nostrils and observe our breath or respiration. The Vipassana is different from pranayama in a sense we follow natural breath here, whereas, in pranayama, the breath is controlled wherein one takes a deep breath and stops for some time; one exhales and stops for some time. The benefit of Vipassana is for the mind, while pranayama is good for the body. Vipassana is a mental exercise to keep the mind healthy, which is much more critical. The body may be very healthy, yet we can't keep our body healthy if our mind is not healthy.

While meditation, we are free to change to the sitting position that suits us. We should, of course, try to keep the back and neck straight. The rhythm of our respiration is the sole object of our concentration. S N Goenkaji, who introduced Vipassana in India, says "Observe the breath diligently, ardently, patiently but persistently and continuously". Then after three days of observing the respiration, one is ready for the second most crucial phase of meditation: "Vipassana", which will be taught on the 4[th]day "Adhithasana" or "the day of strong determination". This time the concentration is not on respiration alone. But all parts of the body from the top of the head to the tip of the toe. We have to sit like a statue one hour every three times a day, without moving our hands and legs. Then only, one may experience different sensations, acute, painful, some lighter-until it becomes like a flow of heat, cold and vibrations in the whole body. But we should not react to pains. Sometimes people have to undergo this 10-day course 4-5 times to detect vibrations. A kind of radiation takes place from person to person, which is a scientific fact today. Since breath is from birth to death for any human being, it is accepted by all as a universal technique. There are no idols or rites, or rituals involved in this meditation. The course is based on the enlightenment of Buddha, which are a) the universality of suffering, b) craving as the root cause of suffering, c) detachment as the remedy for craving d) technique to acquire detachment.

The final aim of meditation is not the concentration of mind but purification by eradicating all mental negativity within. This technique is divided into three parts. A) Sila or moral conduct. Anyone who wishes to practice Vipassana should begin first, practising 'Sila'-ethical or moral conduct., i.e., abstain from killing any creature; stealing; lying; sexual misconduct; taking intoxicants; eating afternoon; body decoration; using substances any luxury beds. However, relaxation is allowed for new students from the last three precepts or those with medical problems. B) Samadhi-mental discipline through concentration of mind C) Panna or wisdom or condition for liberation acquired through "Vipassana". Since 1969, Sri S.N.Goenkaji has been teaching this practice to the world.

At the Vipassana course:

When I published one article in May 2001 in a journal titled "Prayers of world's greatest religions and their symbols", I never thought I would meditate with people of all faiths coming from different parts of the globe very soon. Hindus, Muslims, Christians, Jews, Jains, Parsees, Sikhs and Buddhists and so on. Nearly 300 of us were all together under one roof to become better human beings to practise Vipassana.

When I received the confirmation letter for 10- day Vipassana Course, 5-16 November, 2001 from Vipassana International Academy (VIA) Dhammagiri, Igatpuri, on October 2ndweek, I had mixed feelings. Since I required 12 days leave at short notice. I had to report by 4 PM on 5 November (considered Day-Zero) and would be allowed to leave Dhamma Giri only on 16 November by 7 AM. The letter also said that I should bring bed sheets, blankets, a torch, and enough medicine stock if required during the course. It was also mentioned that laundry service would be available at the Academy during the course.

The letter also said that the participants have to adhere to the code of discipline during the course very carefully. The most important of which are 1) To maintain complete silence from the beginning till Day-10 of the course. 2) To set aside all other meditation practices, rites, rituals, recitations and prayers 3)To maintain complete segregation of sexes 4)to abstain from using any intoxicants, alcohols, tobacco etc. 5)shorts, half pants and transparent clothes are not permitted on the campus.

Igatpuri is a town on central railway 137 km from Mumbai, just 3 hours train journey and 50 km from Nashik. Dhammagiri is just 15 minutes walk from the Igatpuri railway station.

I had to pass several counters supervised by volunteers wearing the batch "DHAMMA WORKER" at the reception. I had to sign a paper agreeing to adhere to the rules of the campus. Finally, I was given an Identity Card which contained my registration number, the room allotted, laundry service, a pouch to put our valuables to be deposited. The card also advised depositing reading and writing materials, talisman, rosary, sacred thread, rudraksha mala, yantra-tantra mala, all electronic gadgets, intoxicants like alcoholic beverages, drugs, tobacco etc. Since my wife reminded me while leaving the house, I had left my holy thread and rudraksha mala at home; hence I had only some cash and credit card to deposit.

At 7:00 PM, the course teacher asked our language preference, whether Hindi or English, for the discourses, and I opted for English. He also briefed me about the course schedule and the code of conduct. Later, we were taken to one of the Dhamma Meditation Halls, where seats were allotted on the floor.

The floor mats consisted of three-inch-thick foam cushions, and we had to pin our slip containing our names, and we were told not to change the seat till the end of the course. Of course, there were few chairs for the students with problems like backache and old age. The group consisted of 18-year youth to 85 years old grandpas coming from all sections of society and professions from near and far around the globe. They were from all walks of life, industrialists, millionaires, executives, farmers, technocrats, doctors, scientists, labourers, judges, addicts, etc. (This fact I came to know only at the end of the course). Later, we were told to assemble in the hall for meditation the next day (Day-1) by 4:30 AM.

Afterwards, I went to my room, where already another participant had occupied his bench. We had to share the bathrooms and toilets with other students. We, roommates, could not talk and look at each other as a rule does not permit. Before retiring, I once again glanced at the daily timetable, which was as follows. 04:00 AM wake up bell; 04:30-06:30 meditation in hall or residence; 06:30-08:00 breakfast ; 09:00-11:00 meditation in hall or residence; 11:00-12:00 lunch; 12:00-01:00 rest;01:00-02:30 meditation in hall or residence; 02:30-03:30 Group meditation in hall; 03:30-05:00 meditation in hall or residence; 05:00-06:00 Tea break; 06:-07:00 Group meditation in hall; 07:00-08:30 Dhamma video discourse by Sri.S.N.Goenkaji; 08:30-09:00 Group meditation in hall;0900:-09:30 Question time in hall; 09:30 retire to room . Light out.

However, we were advised that it is always better to meditate in the hall instead of alone in residence. Accordingly, I meditated in the hall only. The students are kept busy right from 4:30 AM till 9:30 PM. The day starts with a morning wake up bell coming from a giant bell of four feet in length. The bell will be beaten with a wooden log by the guard as per the above timetable. Every bell has its meaning. Students will be eagerly waiting, especially for breakfast, lunch and snack bells. Sitting cross-legged keeping our spine straight for 10 hours a day is painful, but this endurance only builds our self-confidence to face reality in life. In its simplest form, Vipassana is an awareness of our breathing process, which is already an autonomous function of our body. We are living organisms until the time we are breathing. Constant attention on the incoming and outgoing breath is the trick employed to bring us into a relaxed state of mind.

On Day 1: We have to take refuge in the triple Gems in Buddha, Dhamma and Sangha. By doing so, we are not taking refuge in any person, dogma or sect but in Buddha who discovered the path to enlightenment, in the path to reach enlightenment (Dhamma) and in all these saintly persons (monks) who got enlightenment (Sangha). Further, one also has to surrender to the teacher and the course's discipline and timetable. The course is designed based on the experience of thousands of previous students. Day-10 is called Metta day. Today, the technique is taught to fill the mind with thoughts of love, compassion and goodwill for others and world peace.

Dhamma Giri –Igatpuri :

With its lush green, serene and sacred place, the campus is full of various fruit trees, shade trees, including Bodhi (peepal) tree under which the Buddha got enlightenment, flowering shrubs, bushes, climbers and creepers. Since the purchase of this hillock in 1974, thousands of Vipassana Meditators came to meditate and gave their help in establishing the centre. The whole campus of 72 acres has been developed (including the purchase) through voluntary donations (both money and voluntary labour) only from the disciples who have purified themselves through Vipassana meditation. How the site for Dhammagiri centre was chosen makes an exciting story.

Now let us listen to Sri Bhojaraj Sancheti of Igatpuri, the principal Trustee of Vipassana International Academy who has been closely connected with Dhammagiri since 1974 with whom I interacted.

"In December, 1973 I attended my first 10 day Vipassana course at Deolali, near to my home at Igatpuri. On the last day I learned by chance that Goenkaji had been looking for a site to start a meditation centre in the area of Mumbai. At once thought came to me that there could not be more suitable location for such centre than Igatpuri. I was eager for the inexhaustible spring of Dhamma to flow from my town. I approached Goenkaji and invited him for a cup of tea at my house on his way back to Mumbai assuring him that I do not take more than five minutes. After much persuasion, he agreed to stop but warned that five minutes do not turn to five hours. When he came to my house I told him that if he could spare some time I could show three sites for the meditation centre around the town. He did not approve the first two sites shown by me. Then immediately I thought of showing the land where the present Dhamma Giri stands. Goenkaji reached the site and within five minutes he decided that this was what he had been looking for. At that moment someone pointed out that a cremation is taking place at the foot of the hill on which we stood. I was worried that the proximity of a cremation ground would change the mind of Goenkaji but he said with a smile "Good". This will continuously implant the awareness of anicca (impermanence) in the mind of meditators".

I learnt that then and there itself, Sri Ragil Mehta, a fellow meditator of Bhojaraj Sancheti, offered to purchase the property and donate it to the Trust. Sri Bhojaraj Sancheti continued to say, "Though five minute really turned to five hours, that day-

December16, 1973. It was the happiest day of my life. Since then I have practiced Vipassana faithfully and given whatever free time I have to serve the Dhamma so that many may experience liberation."

Today, Dhamma Giri stands like a Jewel in the mountainous landscape. On one side Igatpuri town and all other sides we find paddy fields and behind rock mountains. There would be many waterfalls during the monsoon. The view from Dhamma Giri is enchanting and makes an ideal meditation centre. The main attraction of Dhamma Giri is the Pagoda constructed in 1979.

During 10- day course, participants remain within the campus, having no contact with outside the world. One had to stay silent without having access to T.V., Radio, newspapers, or mobile calls. They have to refrain from reading, writing and suspend any religious or other practices like Yoga. Some participants run away in the middle of the course on the pretext of ill health or cannot adhere to the code of conduct.

Dhamma Giri is a world within a world. It provides comfortable residences for 700 students with wholesome vegetarian food.—spacious halls for group meditation and individual cells for individual meditation. There are separate building reception offices, book stores, male course offices, female course offices, and teachers' residences. A large kitchen complex uses modern appliances and caters to over 900 people daily. Male and female areas are restricted within the complex, and female Dhamma Workers guard the female area. The essential rule is to maintain noble silence, which means the silence of body and speech. Even glancing, gestures and direct eye contact among the students during Day-1 to Day- 9 are prohibited. However, students can talk to Asst. Teachers and Dhamma Workers if the need arises.

The food is also excellent under self -service system. The breakfast at 6:30 consists of items like poha (beaten rice), idli, dhokla, saboo daana kichdi, sweet porridge (Shira), brown bread, half cup of tea or a full cup of milk. Sugarless porridge, tea and milk were available for people with diabetes. Lunch at 11:00AM consists of normal vegetarian Gujarati or Maharashtrian style meals and boiled vegetables and green vegetables. There was no dinner. It was only a snack at 5:00 PM consisting of two bananas or two loose skinned oranges and a little kurkure(puffed rice) with half a cup of tea or whole milk. Even this banana is not served for old students, but only lemon water. However, on health grounds, old students can have fruits.

The principle here is that student has to lead the life of a monk or nun. The food is like a biksha or alms where monks take food given as charity by old Vipassana students. The dining hall is so big that all the 300 participants could finish their meals within half an hour without any hassle. Different kinds of water, say filtered water, hot water, hot ginger water, an ordinary drinking water, were available 24 hours a day in the dining hall. Hot water was also open from 6:30-7:30 AM for the bath. The male meditation hall is so big that it can accommodate 350 people on the floor on cushions. There would be pin-drop silence except for the sound of chirping birds, squirrels, wind breeze and bells from Pagoda top.

Since everyone has to maintain "noble silence"-that is, the silence of body, speech and mind in Dhamma Giri, as a means of communication, the campus has hundreds of signboards that display notices in Hindi and English. Still, every one of them bears and "Be happy" at the end in small fonts. At every convenient location, there are drinking water facilities and urinals. All areas of the campus are not permitted for students during the course. Hence we find boards like "No 10 Day students beyond this point", "Only 30/45 days students", "Female area", "No male students beyond this area", "No students beyond this point", etc. Even when the vow of silence is broken on Day 10 at 10:00 AM, males are not allowed to the female area vice versa. In other words, the husband and wife attending the course on the campus can talk only on Day-10 only, near the dining hall or gate. Near the drinking water area board says, "Please do not touch the glass to your lips". Whether dining hall, meditation hall, discourse hall, or Pagoda (chaitya), shoes stand where footwear must be removed and kept. There are separate queues for an evening snack in the dining hall itself, one for the new students and the other for the old students. Since senior students are supposed to take only lemon water. Silence is observed for the first nine full days. On the tenth day, one can resume speech to re-establish the regular pattern of daily life. Continuity of practice is the secret of success in this course, and hence silence is an essential component in maintaining this continuity.

A previous student gives each student who attends a Vipassana course this gift. There is no charge for either the teaching or for room and board. All Vipassana courses worldwide are run on a strictly voluntary donations (Daana) basis. At the end of your course, if one finds benefit from the experience, you are welcome to donate for the coming course, according to your volition and means. The teachers also give Vipassana purely as a service to others. All they get is the satisfaction of seeing people's happiness at the end of ten days.

A student taking a Vipassana course practices renounces the householders' responsibilities for the course duration. They live like a monk or a nun, on the charity of others. It reduces the ego, a significant cause of their misery. It is another reason. If one even pays a small token fee, then the ego gets built up, and one may say, "Oh, I want this. This facility is not to my liking", " I can do whatever I want here", and so on. This ego becomes a significant hindrance in progressing on the path of Dhamma. It is another reason why a fee is not charged. This has been the Dhamma tradition for millennia.

Dhamma Workers: I should say something about "Dhamma Workers", who are all old students and who also came at their cost from far and near for ten days self-less service for the spread of Vipassana-Dhamma, inspired by Sri Goenkaji. While young chap Mr Oren came from New Jersey, USA, the other came from Israel, who did all sorts of errand jobs whether at the reception, dining hall, meditation hall or discourse, laundry counter etc. They are all of different age groups, and according to the age group, the work is assigned. The wake-up service in the morning is very humorous to observe. Even after 04:30 AM who do not wake up, the Dhamma Worker will go outside the room making a sound with a small two-inch bell until they get up or those who loiter before the meditation hall until they go inside the hall.

Later, on Day-10, I learned that there were 330 males and 250 females for this course, including around 30 foreign nationals from countries like Mexico, U.S., UK, Israel, Iran, Germany, Italy, Korea, Sri Lanka, Thailand and Japan. I learnt that there were one group of 12 ladies from Iran for whom there were separate discourses in the Persian language. On Day-10, there was a video show "Islands of Dhamma", a documentary film on centres of Vipassana meditation around the world.

Though World Teacher of Vipassana Sri S.N.Goenkaji will always be on tour to spread Vipassana, he reaches students through his audios and videos while Assistant Teachers conduct the courses. Nearly 100,000 students are trained in meditation throughout the world in a year. The exciting thing is, neither Teacher S.N.Goenkaji nor Asst. Teachers (Nearly 600 worldwide) receive any remuneration. Further, the centres worldwide (now nearly 200 centres and 150 non-centres) do not charge any fees for the course. Expenses for the food and lodging are all met by voluntary donations of old students who experienced the benefit of Vipassana, wish to give others the same opportunity. In this way, each meditator lives on gratitude and charity of an old student for 10 days.

Further, throughout the globe, the centres have been developed through donations, including land purchase. We have to learn from S.N.Goenkaji that nowhere his name or photo appears on the campus. I felt that is the reason he inspires the students. Irrespective of the country, caste, colour, economic status, everybody is treated alike on the campus.

Goenkaji says, "When the misery is a universal malady, the remedy cannot be sectarian. It also must be universal. Awareness of one's respiration meets this requirement. Human actions are of mind and body. The mind constantly tries to escape from the present reality and moves into the past and future that is not attainable, and therefore this wild mind remains agitated. Vipassana technique is an art of living on which one can live only in the present. Hence, the first step to learn to be present in reality is to observe our breath, which results in the concentration of mind. Nobody else can do the job for us. One has to work hard for oneself to get liberated. It leaves no room for miseries, shortcuts or dependency on any "Guru". On Day-10, by 10:00 AM, the students can exchange views with fellow students when silence is broken. The counters for receiving donations and selling publications were also opened on this day. I purchased some books and subscribed to the monthly Vipassana Newsletter. I also donated cash with gratitude.

Vipassana is taught in many prisons, police training colleges, the corporate world, including some management schools. Some state governments give paid leave to their officers and staff to attend this course. Already reputed companies like IPCL, Mahindra, ONGC etc., encourage their employees to participate in this course. IAS training academy, Mussoorie also teaches Vipassana.

A Vipassana meditator has to keep in mind that one has to follow ten mental perfections in one's daily life; otherwise, it will not give the desired results. They are renunciation, morality, effort and forbearance, adherence to truth, strong determination, wisdom, equanimity, selfless love and charity. Though man may find it difficult to adhere, the world would be different even if one tries to go on this path. In Buddha's time, there was peace everywhere, and everything was in plenty because the needs were kept at a bare minimum. The edicts of Emperor Ashoka (one of the largest empires in the world then) also reveal that he and his vast sections of his people practised Vipassana.

We were allowed entry into the Pagoda on Day-10. I felt it was a wonderful experience that helped me to cleanse my body, mind and soul. We should be proud that the tree of Dhamma has begun spreading its branches in the land of its roots.

How did Vipassana lose to India?

The Siddhartha Gautam, the Buddha, attained enlightenment at the age of 35, the true happiness of liberation (free from mental defilements and rebirths) and also discovered this Vipassana technique and distributed with compassion throughout the remaining years of his life, till his nirvana(passing away) at the age of 80. However, India lost this excellent technique within 500 years due to mixing it with different rites, rituals, philosophical beliefs, etc. After some time, those rituals and ideas became more attractive to people than Vipassana itself and slowly lost their efficacy and disappeared from the land of its origin. Fortunately, the neighbouring country Burma (present Myanmar) preserved the original through millennia. The Bhikkhu Sangha of Myanmar held the scriptures. The Buddha said, "Rare is human life, rare to encounter the Dhamma (Law of Nature), we are fortunate to have both; let us work to banish suffering". The technique of Vipassana offers equal benefit to all who practice it without any discrimination based on race, class or sex. Benefits are proportionate to the extent of the practice. But confronting realities about oneself is not so easy. In Vipassana practice, there is no memory involved. It is awareness of mind and matter within the framework of the body along with wisdom.

Sri S.N.Goenkaji-The torchbearer of Vipassana to the World:

Sri S.N.Goenkaji(1924), a native of Burma(present Myanmar), taught Vipassana in India and World. Though Goenkaji claims to teach what Buddha taught, he does not call himself a Buddhist. Temples, monasteries, churches and mosques have hosted his meditation retreats, and hundreds of Christian priests and nuns have also attended the Vipassana course.

Sri Goenkaji was born in a wealthy merchant family and succeeded in the business at a very young age. But the success brought with it "a lot of tension," as he put it, and he began to suffer from severe migraine headache. The best doctors in Burma could not cure him except by giving morphine injections. Afraid of becoming an addict, Goenkaji sought medical care in the best hospitals in Europe, America and Japan but to no avail. Upon returning to Burma in 1955, a friend suggested he take a 10-day Vipassana course with Sayagi U B.Khin. Besides being a meditation master, he held a high position in the government as an Accountant General of Burma.

"I was hesitant initially", Goenkaji recalls, "partly because I could not believe this meditation could help me when best doctors in the world could not do it. Partly because it was Buddhist course and I came from a very staunch Hindu family. But meeting him changed my mind". After attending the Vipassana course, Sri Goenkaji got relief from his migraine and the stress and tension of the business. He practised Vipassana with Sayagi U B.Khin for the next fourteen years, and Sri Goenkaji was authorised as Vipassana Teacher in 1969. He also studied Pali and became a scholar in the Buddha's language, and his teachings (the Dhamma) have been preserved.

Sayagi had a strong belief in the prophecy that the Vipassana-Dhamma would arise once again 2500 years after the time of Buddha, in the land of Buddha and from there, it would spread around the world, serving the suffering humanity at large. He often used to say, 'Burma owes a great debt to India which must be repaid". His prediction has come true today.

Sri. Goenkaji returned to India, due to the persuasion of Sayagi, as his representative in 1969. Along with him, the Vipassana technique and the entire available Pali literature. The first Vipassana course in India was conducted in Mumbai on 3 July 1969. Since then, he has been spreading Vipassana both in India and abroad. India should be ever grateful to Sayagi U B.Khin, who passed away in 1971.

This teacher (Guruji) Sri Goenkaji has no beard, long hair, ochre robes, or marks on the forehead. He is modern and very ordinary in the dress. He is married to Mrs Ilaichi Devi, and they have six sons, most of whom live together in a traditional joint family house in Mumbai.

Goenkaji is a poet and an outstanding orator. His melodic voice in Pali, in his daily chanting, brings a wave of love, compassion and goodwill towards all beings. The course participants long remember the narration of stories, his smile, laughter and sense of humour during his daily Dhamma discourse. Some of the stories are from events in the life of the Buddha, Indian folk tales and the personal experiences of Sri Goenkaji. The stories lighten the serious atmosphere of the Vipassana course and bring inspiration to the students every day.

Goenkaji has given much time and importance in recent years for Pali studies. The Vipassana International Academy (VRI) was established under his guidance to research both theory and practice of the Buddha's teachings. Sri S.N.Goenkaji is one of the few Indian spiritual leaders who never sought publicity, preferring to relay in word of mouth to spread interest in Vipassana. He always emphasised the importance of actual meditation practice over mere writings about meditation. Sri S.N.Goenkaji says, "Every life is a preparation for the next death if someone is wise he or she will use this life to best advantage and prepare for a good death".

Goenkaji says, "According to our karmas of the past, the flow of our life goes in a particular direction—miserable or happy, whatever it is. This is because of our own karmas; nobody else has created this. Whatever you have done in your past is gone; you can't help it. But today you are your own master. With your present practice, you can change the entire flow. So destiny can be changed. You are your own master, the master of your present. Truth is God. Realise the truth within you, and you will realise God. We observe our own breath because breath is a true fact. It is the truth that is closely associated not only with our body but also with our mind. Respiration is related not only to the body but to the mind as well. When we breathe in, the lungs get inflated with air and when we breathe out, the lungs are deflated. This is how the respiration is related to the body. If an impurity arises in the mind, the normal pace of the breath gets disturbed. This is how respiration is related to the mind." Moreover, this knowledge should be experiential rather than what we tell or study in books, etc. We have started this practise of observing the breath.

Vipassana Meditator does not become "A Buddhist":

Siddhartha Gautama, the Buddha, neither taught Buddhism nor converted a single person "a Buddhist" during his lifetime. The word Buddha stands for any enlightened person. Buddha taught was Dhamma(Dharma), the truth, the universal law of nature and inspired millions of people to follow it. It is proved that in the entire ancient literature of Buddha's teachings, commentaries and sub commentaries, amongst a total of 52,602 pages containing 74,48,248 words, the word of Buddha is absent. He gave 82000 discourses during his lifetime. Those who followed the teachings of Buddha were never called "Buddhist" during his period. We do not know when, where, by whom and why the use of the words "Buddhism" and "Buddhist" started. One research at International Vipassana Academy, Igatpuri, also reveals that until about 500 years after Buddha, the word "Buddha " was not found in any ancient spiritual literature of India. The Academy also says it needs further research.

It is most important to know that Buddha's teachings are not limited to any particular religion. His teachings are universal and non-sectarian. Dhamma (Buddha's teachings) is the most precious legacy ancient India gave to the world. The Dhamma is the applicable code of conduct, a way of purity and gracious living. They are the scientific study of the mind and the matter and ultimate truth. The Buddha should be considered a super scientist who studied the fundamental law of nature governing the universe by direct personal experience.

The unique feature of Buddha's teachings is that he did not merely give sermons but gave practical technique "Vipassana" to help people achieve this. Millions of people followed him in his period and led a contented and happy life. When Christian's higher authorities of the Roman Catholic Order convinced that the practice of Vipassana is a non-sectarian and suitable for all, permitted to attend the course, this opened the gate for hundreds of Christian priests and nuns to join the course both in India and abroad. According to Sri S.N.Goenkaji, the regular practice of about two hours per day helps develop our potentialities and become better human beings. It helps us to radiate love and compassion to wish happiness to the whole world.

Developments in science, technology, transportation, communication, agriculture and medicine have revolutionised human life at the material level. But this is only superficial: underneath modern men and women are living in conditions of great mental and emotional stress, even in developed and affluent countries.

The problems and conflicts arising out of racial, ethnic, sectarian and caste prejudice affect the citizens of every country. People everywhere are eager to find a method that can bring peace and harmony. Vipassana is the only way to transform the human mind and character. The opportunity is awaiting all those who sincerely wish to make an effort.

Daily meditation brings peace of mind, which ultimately improves our efficiency in day-to-day life. The benefit of Vipassana in day to day life summarised:

Concentration on the breath helps to live in the present and not in the past or future and be in equanimity accepting all outcomes be it good or bad. By maintaining specific postures and noble silence, we develop the self-discipline to lead a happy and healthy life. The principle of Anicca-everything will pass away one day (the law of impermanence) will also be experienced in the observance of the sensations in the body. It will help to develop the tranquillity of mind towards changing realities. During the course, we consistently reminded that all of the people in our lives and our possessions, including ourselves, grow old and die one day. It helps to become more compassionate, loving and generate goodwill towards all beings; the method of meditation is more experiential than intellectual; More than anything else, Vipassana is the art of becoming a better human being. Goenkaji says, "There is only one place to find real peace, real harmony. That place is within".

Studies have established its beneficial role as a positive mental health measure in various psychosomatic disorders, personality disorders, besides alcohol and drug abuse & addiction. Numerous anecdotal case reports of persons suffering from various health disorders, both physical and mental, are available, pointing out the therapeutic efficacy of Vipassana. Besides, the technique has found ready acceptance with the healers of diverse disciplines, such as Yoga, Naturopathy, Homeopathy, Ayurveda, Allopathy, etc., as it is free from dogmas, based on experience and focussed on relief from human suffering. However, it is to emphasise that any such health benefit is considered just a by-product of this profound technique of mental purification. The practice of Vipassana does hasten the healing process, but more importantly, it transforms one's approach to life and its vicissitudes. One learns to face all sickness and suffering with equanimity; the healers augment their ability to be a professional anchor to the sick in the tumult of their lives.

Research conducted at the All India Institute of Medical Sciences has established that Vipassana meditation increases persons' control of their emotions, reducing feelings of anger, tension, hostility, revenge, and helplessness. Drug addiction, neurotic and psychopathological symptoms also get diminished. In addition, prison inmates practising Vipassana meditation have shown an increased willingness to work, participate in other treatment programmes, abide by prison rules, and co-operate with prison authorities. The striking example of Dhamma Tihar, New Delhi, has attracted many prisons worldwide to use Vipassana meditation as a tool for rehabilitation. The study conducted under the auspices of the University of Washington indicates a significant decrease in the re-offence of the jail inmates practising Vipassana. The Jail Personnel of the North Rehabilitation Facility (NRF) in Seattle, Washington, found that those who complete the Vipassana course are calmer, better disciplined and more reasonable. All these researches show that Vipassana is now practised in prisons in the USA, Spain, Mexico, Thailand, Taiwan, and New Zealand.

Professionals in the private sector and Government officials facing stressful lifestyles attend the Vipassana course. Many management institutes like Symbiosis and Sadhana Institute of Pune have made the 10-day Vipassana course a part of their curriculum. The Government of Maharashtra has been a pioneer in introducing Vipassana to State Government officials since 1996. Since 2003, the government has been granting commuted leave of 14 days to attend a Vipassana course to all state government employees. Organisations such as Maharashtra State Electricity Board (MSEB), Yashwantrao Chavan Academy of Development Administration (YASHADA), Pune have also followed suit. The Government of Maharashtra has included the courses for children in its Mumbai schools as part of the activity.

After this, I attended two more 10-day Vipassana courses in 2005 at Dhamma Siri, South West Vipassana Centre, Kaufman, Texas, U.S. and the other in 2017 at Dhamma Paphulla, Bangalore. Whenever time permits, I sit for meditation since the benefits are immense in gaining strong willpower to maintain a medicine-free life. Attending repeated Vipassana meditation courses helped me develop more self-confidence, manage stress and lead a peaceful life.

Acharya Goenkaji's had most fervent Dhamma wanted to establish a Global Vipassana Pagoda[2] in Mumbai, which was fulfilled in November 2008 when the construction was completed. The massive inner dome seats over 8000 people. The pagoda complex aims to express gratitude to Gautama Buddha for dispensing universal teaching for the eradication of suffering, to reveal the truth about the life of Buddha and His teaching, and to provide a place for the practice of Vipassana meditation. He hoped that this monument would bridge different communities, sects, countries, and races to make the world a more harmonious and peaceful.

Sri S.N.Goenka was conferred the Padma Bhushan award in 2012. Shri S.N.Goenka passed away in Mumbai on 29 September 2013, but he continues to teach Vipassana Meditation through audios and videos assisted by Assistant Teachers throughout the world in all centres.

CHAPTER TEN

Possessing Natural Doctors

One cannot buy eternal happiness through wealth. Good health and longevity are the domain of the individual body. People have to take care of their bodies with the discipline of the mind. Enthusiasm and cheerfulness for work is good health which comes through compassion for fellow human beings. Anger and hate is the real cause for stress. If we fall ill, the immediate impact of the illness would be on our family. Nature has bestowed human beings with many means to prevent or cure different kinds of diseases. The day we are born count down starts for our death. No one is immortal or infinite. According to the National Council on Ageing (NCOA), about 92 per cent of seniors have at least one chronic disease, and 77 per cent have at least two.[1] Hypertension, Heart disease, brain stroke, diabetes and cancer are among the most common and costly chronic health conditions causing two-thirds of deaths each year in the United States. India is also stepping into the same situation. It is better to have a holistic approach to lead a healthy lifestyle.

Among many, I consider the following things as Preventive Medicines- The Natural Doctors: Self-confidence (willpower), sleep, sun, diet, exercise and friends. These six doctors can have a significant impact on our health without any financial burden. They help to postpone morbidity. These possesssions are also complementary to any medical system, say Western medicine, homoeopathy, Ayurveda etc. Sometimes they act as self-healing mechanisms in the body both physically and psychologically. Of course, these are not evidence-based therapies but create a strong foundation for curing any disease. The advantage is they strengthen body immunity and reduce the risk of chronic diseases. Our aim should be to keep cheerful and happy till the last breath. Can you imagine the pain we have to bear if we get treatment in hospitals as patients with a given number during registration? I will explain the levels or stages of our treatment in any hospital. Hospitals have different categories of patients and depending on the severity of the diseases. They keep us in the respective units, say Outpatient department (OPD), Emergency Units (EU), Critical care units (CCU), High Dependency Units (HCU), Operation rooms (OR), Intensive care units (ICU) without ventilators, ICU with ventilators. Natural doctors give us the power to avoid going to any of these units under public or private hospitals in our country.

Henry Miller (1891-1980), an American writer and artist, wrote, "Develop an interest in life as you see it; the people, the things, literature, music- the world is so rich, simply throbbing with rich treasures; beautiful souls and interesting people. Forget yourself."

In this context, here I also present a beautiful poem by Pablo Neruda (1904-1973), a Nobel Prize winner for literature in 1971, a masterpiece philosophy of life. He left a rich legacy for the coming generation. Pablo was a Chilean poet, once called the greatest poet of the 20th century in any language.

"You start dying slowly

If you do not travel,

If you do not read,

If you do not listen to sounds of life,

If you do not appreciate yourself.

You start dying slowly

When you kill your self-esteem,

When you do not let others help you.

You start dying slowly

If you become a slave to your habits,
Walking every day on the same paths.....,
If you do not change your routine,
If you do not wear different colours
Or you do not speak to those you don't know.
You start dying slowly
If you avoid feeling the passion
And its turbulent emotions;
Those which make your eyes glisten
And your heartbeat fast.
You start dying slowly.
If you do not change your life when you are not
Satisfied with your job, or with your love,
If you do not risk what is safer for the uncertain,
If you do not go after your dream,
If you do not allow yourself
At least once in your lifetime,
To run away from sensible advice....."
-Pablo Neruda

The poem's theme is that life becomes meaningful when we follow our passion, make new friends, increase our knowledge, face unique challenges, see new places, wear new dresses and chase new dreams. When we lose our self-esteem, get afraid of taking risks, keep doing something repeatedly, we start dying slowly. It describes the beauty of life, and every line is the gospel of wisdom.

No one can contribute to our health as much we can. Everyone in the chosen profession begins with hopes and aspirations. But all dreams never materialise to which we need not worry. The leading cause of any disease is fear, depression, anxiety, stress or tension. Stress reduces body immunity by 40 per cent, as established by studies. Even our annual body check-up recommended by doctors or health professionals is also due to fear only. Indian Council of Medical Research recommends regularly checking for blood sugar, lipids and blood pressure after

30 years at least every six months. You may call me an odd person because I do not believe in this annual blood test and body check-up as long as I feel illness of any kind. I remember the animals like cattle, dogs or cats who observe fast during fever or when they feel uneasy and get cured naturally. If we think more about our body and blood, we end up with more confusion and fear psychosis.

Similarly, I feel that nature will take care if we give little time to heal. Western medicine offers a cure, but they have a long list of side effects. But these things are not discussed with the patients they have prescribed. Under this context, nature provides a sound solution. It is a proven fact that when one is in close communion with nature, one can be happy, healthy and content.

Thanks to the medical fraternity who have found several vaccines, drugs and medical procedures that helped raise the life expectancy in the developed world from 45 in the 20th century to 79 in the 21st century, adding nearly 34 years over one century. Many contagious diseases are eradicated. However, nowadays, the medical profession has become a big business but with few exceptions. In many remote villages well qualified private medical practitioners offer primary health service at doorsteps with compassion and dedication, charging very nominal fees. Mother Nature has given us choice to become self- doctor without any side effects. If we follow the six natural self-healing doctors, I am sure we will save money and avoid going to hospitals as a patient.

High blood pressure or hypertension was not considered a disease till recently. Still, nowadays, it is the leading cause of damage to the heart, kidney, brain, thyroid and eyes and related organs. Life is not worth living means going into depression and loneliness. Because of improvement in medical facilities and regular medication, people can feel that diseases appear to be cured, but the ageing process will continue. The medicines only have pushed the death. Earlier deaths used to be in homes, but now it is in the hospitals. I consider death at home would be peaceful. At least we need not go through the treatment by a battery of doctors, specialists and super-specialists. But dying in the hospital is common now.

Further, when age advances, the patient's decisions about treatments are taken by their kin. Becoming a patient in the hospital is the most fearful thing for a healthy person. In the fourteenth century philosophy, the word patient meant "the object of an action". The fundamental truth is that all organisms die and strive for one or the other issue until their last breath.

Nobody is aware of what happens at the last stage of death because very few writers or doctors could document their death experience or nearer to the end. However, here I describe two American doctors; surprisingly, both have an Indian connection. Paul Kalanithi, whose mother was an Indian born, penned a book, "When breath becomes air", his own death experience. Atul Gawande, whose father an Indian born, wrote a book "Being mortal, medicine and what matters in the end" on advanced ageing and death experience of his elderly patients, including his father.

Everybody is sure they will die one day, but nobody knows when and what form death comes—a mystery of life. But Paul Kalanithi (April 11, 1977 –March 9, 2015) knew it almost accurately. He was Stanford University neurosurgical chief resident who was to become a brain surgeon in later years. In May 2013, twenty-two months before his death Paul Kalanithi was diagnosed with Stage IV metastatic lung cancer. Six months before his diagnosis of cancer, he started losing weight and having severe back pain. He was told an 80 per cent chance of death within two years. Then he started documenting his experience till the last minute of fighting with death in hospital. Brain surgeons, also known as neurosurgeons, perform complex surgeries on the brain, spinal cord, and peripheral nerves. They must possess a medical degree, complete a neurosurgery residency, and obtain state licensing. Job growth for all surgeons is faster than average and highest-paid doctors anywhere in the world. Brain surgeons examine, diagnose, and surgically treat disorders of the nervous system.

Training to become a brain surgeon requires a 6-7 year neurosurgical residency following four years of medical school. Still, qualified brain surgeons receive some of the highest salaries of all medical health professionals. This career is physically and intellectually demanding and requires excellent hand dexterity and hand-eye coordination. Paul Kalanithi, at thirty-six, had reached the pinnacle of the mountain top. In the following year, his residency would have ended. Paul always treated his patients with empathy and compassion. He had won prestigious national awards and was getting job offers from several major universities. But death always wins. He conducted several very difficult neurosurgeries but became a terminal lung cancer patient in the same hospital at Stanford.

Paul Kalanithi wrote, "I was transferred to the ICU. Part of my soft palate and pharynx died from dehydration and peeled out of my mouth. I was in pain, floating through varying levels of consciousness, while a pantheon of specialists was brought together to help: medical intensivists (critical care physician), nephrologists, gastroenterologists, endocrinologists, infectious disease specialists, neurosurgeons, general oncologists, thoracic oncologists, otolaryngologists."

He had a lifelong love for writing and reading. He wrote that the nervous system comprises the central and peripheral nervous systems: The brain and the spinal cord are major nervous systems. The nerves that go through the whole body make up the peripheral nervous system.

He was always curious to know what makes life meaningful. He had taken English and biology major as an undergraduate at Stanford and then stayed on for a Master in English literature. He wrote, "For my thesis, I studied the work of Walt Whitman, a poet who, a century before, was possessed by the same questions that haunted me, who wanted to find a way to understand and describe what he termed "the Physiological-Spiritual Man."

He also earned an MPhil in history and philosophy of science and medicine from the University of Cambridge, and later, he graduated from the Yale School of Medicine. He had a lifelong love for writing and reading. After graduating from medical school, Kalanithi returned to Stanford to complete his residency training in neurosurgery and a postdoctoral fellowship in neuroscience at Stanford University School of Medicine. He died at the age of 38, leaving behind his wife and eight-month-old daughter. Eight months before his death, his daughter was born. Paul's editorial support at the Random House (The publisher) motivated him to complete the book before his end. At that time, the manuscript was just an open file on his computer. Paul asked his family as his dying wish to publish posthumously. His wife, Lucy Kalanithi, fulfilled the wish by writing the last chapter epilogue. That is how we could read his thoughts today.

He understood that the brain gives rise to our ability to form a relationship and make life meaningful. Our brain shielded in a thick centimetre skull relates to passion, hunger, love, digestive tracts, and heartbeat throughout life. If a person is not breathing means, his heartbeat will stop. The capacity of the aged blood to take oxygen from old tissues of the lungs declines over the years. It is part of the ageing process. "Diseases are molecules misbehaving, the basic requirement of life is metabolism and death is cessation".

He wrote, "Where did biology, mortality, literature and philosophy intersect? This is medicine." Though his father, uncle, elder brother, and wife (internist) were all doctors, none could help him survive. He wanted to find out the answer to what makes human life meaningful till we face death and decay. That is why he studied literature, philosophy, science and medicine. His journey from medical student to professor of neurosurgery took him almost ten years of relentless training and internship.

He always carried his laptop even when chemotherapy dripped into his veins. When tarceva oral tablets and chemotherapy had stopped working, he singularly focused on finishing the book within the limited life expectancy in his final months. The manuscript for the book was partially finished, and Paul knew that he was unlikely to complete it as he lost stamina, clarity and time. At the last stage, he expressed a desire to take the oxygen mask off and start morphine to become unconscious and die peacefully. Paul confronted death and accepted it as a physician and patient. He wanted to help people understand death and face their mortality. Paul Kalanithi's book "When breath becomes air" became The New York Times Non-Fiction Best Seller. [2]

Atul Gawande is a surgeon, writer, and public health researcher, practising general and endocrine surgery at Brigham and Women's Hospital in Boston. He wrote a book, "Being Mortal, Medicine and What Matters in the End", covering ageing, frailty or dying. Medical schools teach how to save lives but not how to tend to their demise. In the industrialised world, the experience of advanced ageing and death has shifted to hospitals and nursing homes. Modern scientific capabilities have profoundly altered the course of human life. People live longer and better than at any time in history. But scientific advances have turned the process of ageing and dying into medical experiences matters to be managed by healthcare professionals. He took an interest in the care and treatment of the elderly. He relates his own experiences with patients who had terminal diseases.

He suggests palliative caregivers should focus on removing as much pain and suffering from the patient as possible and finding out what he would like to do with the rest of his life, and trying to help him achieve those aspirations. We accept that we are all ageing and not escaping from the tragedy of life, which is dying one day. The book throws light on the limitations of medicines and living to last breath with freedom, dignity and joy. We should focus less on prolonging life and making it a meaningful good life in twilight years. People who feel not worth living go through depression and loneliness. Many terminal patients say, "Never wake me up again from ICU.I want to die." Doctors are beginning to recognise that not everyone can be cured and that some people need comfort, kindness, attention and understanding and the chance to have a purpose. Death waits for every one of us, but the pathway need not be through misery and a loss of independence and purpose.[3]

Zhou Daxin, a Chinese novelist, wrote a book recently "The Sky Gets Dark Slowly". It is a sensitive exploration of old age and the complex, hidden emotional words of the elderly in a rapidly ageing population. He writes, "Many elders are completely unprepared for what they are to face when it comes to getting old and the road that lays ahead of them". In the time between a person turning 60 years old, as they begin to age, right until all the lights go out and the sky gets dark, there are some situations to keep in mind, so that you will be prepared for what is to come. And you will not panic. 1. The people by your side will only continue to grow smaller in number. People in your parent's side and grandparent's generations have predominantly all left, many of your peers will increasingly find it harder to look after themselves, and the younger generations will all be busy with their own lives. Even your wife or husband may depart earlier than you, then come the days of emptiness. You will have to learn how to live alone and to enjoy and embrace solitude. 2. Society will care less for you. No matter how glorious your previous career was or how famous you are, ageing will continually transform you into a regular older adult and old lady. The spotlight no longer shines on you, and you will have to learn to be content with standing quietly in one corner, to admire and appreciate the hubbub and views that come after you, and you must overcome the urge to be envious or grumble. 3. The road ahead will be rocky and full of precocity. Fractures, cardiovascular blockages, brain atrophy, cancer These are all possible guests that could visit you any time, and you would not be able to turn them away. You will have to live with illness and ailments to view them as friends, do not even fantasise about stable, quiet days without any trouble in your body. Maintaining positivity and getting appropriate and adequate exercise is your duty, and you have to encourage yourself to keep consistency. 4. Prepare for bed-bound life, a return to the infant state. Our mothers brought us into this world on a bed after a life of struggle. We return to our starting point -the bed-and to the state of having to be looked after by others. The only difference is that we once had our mothers to care for us, but when we prepare to leave, we may not even have our kin look after us. Even if we have kin, their care may never come close to that of your mother's. You will more likely be cared for by nursing staff who bear zero relation to you, wearing smiles on their faces while carrying weariness and boredom in their hearts. Lay still, and don't be difficult; remember to be grateful.

Before the sky gets dark, the last stretches of life's journey will gradually get dimmer and dimmer. Naturally, it will be harder to see the path ahead that you are treading towards, and it will be harder to keep going forward. As such, upon turning 60, it would do us all well to see life for what it is, to cherish what we have, to enjoy life whilst we can, and do not take on society's troubles or your children's affairs on for yourself. Stay humble, don't act superior on account of your age and talk down to others-this will hurt yourself as much as it will hurt others. As we get older, all the better, should we understand what respect is and what it counts. In these later days of your lives, you have to understand what it means, let go of your attachments, and mentally prepare yourself. The way of nature is the way of life; go with its flow, and live with equanimity.[4]

Another thing is when we age, we need to take care of our body and imbibe the concept of "I love my body"; "I live for myself"; "I love my food"; "I live independent to my last breath". Independent means here concerning our daily activities without assistance such as shopping, preparing food (if the need arises), maintaining housekeeping, doing our laundry, managing medicines, making mobile calls, travelling, managing finances, maintaining body hygiene, etc. Philanthropically this may look odd because it says we have to live for others, but body fitness is fundamental to our life. If we are ill and bedridden, we are a liability to our kin. We come alone and also leave this world alone one day. The doctors say it is essential to control risk factors like cholesterol, blood sugar, obesity and blood pressure to avoid chronic diseases later, including cancer.

According to a study conducted using 453854 fasting blood sugar samples across five cities-Ahmedabad, Bengaluru, Chennai, Kochi and Hyderabad-by Neuberg Diagnostics found that 24 per cent of the people were pre-diabetic or borderline diabetic. Sujay Prasad, Neuberg Diagnostics, said "Before becoming diabetic a healthy person goes through a stage of pre-diabetes, lasting a few months to a couple of years, depending on lifestyle and diet. During the pre-diabetes stage the blood sugar is elevated but not enough to satisfy the international criteria. This awareness will help persons with pre-diabetes manage sugar levels and prevent them from becoming diabetic. Pre-diabetes can develop at any age, however with advanced age, the risk becomes higher." There are no symptoms in pre-diabetes, which makes it as much of a silent killer as diabetes. It can be reversed with diet, exercise and weight loss provided the person does not gain the weight back. "Blood sugar from food needs to be pushed into muscles, liver and fat which is done by insulin. But when there is too much blood sugar it spills into blood. The body produces more and more insulin while organs develop insulin resistance. Excess blood sugar then settles around the belly. This leads to fatty liver in men and polycystic ovarian disease (PCOD) in women. Insulin resistance leads to weight gain". Organs such as kidney, eyes as well as the nervous system cannot resist insulin and then get affected.

If we keep the six natural doctors, we are sure to overcome medication or hospitalisation. As far as I am concerned I continue to undertake all the activities required to maintain medicine free life. Further I drive both two wheelers and four wheelers even long distances keeping the natural doctors for the sake of my body. I normally ignore minor variations in my health parameters and avoid taking medicines immediately.

The natural doctors are described here below.

Natural Doctor No.1. Self-Confidence:

It is a fact that our ability to ward off diseases depends on how our immune system exists. While our immune system is genetic, staying healthy depends on our lifestyle. Immunity is like a fortress and sets up several lines of defence against diseases. Our body can fight infections and stay fit. All of us are born with antibodies that work as a strong shield against diseases. However, each one of us has a different reaction to certain diseases. For example: If we are immune to colds, we may not be resistant to malaria. Our immunity levels are made differently. It is called our natural immunity. Dr. B M Hegde, popularly known as a people's doctor and most significant proponent of preventive medicines and home remedies, says, "Healing is done by our own immune system not by any surgery or medicine". Passive immunity is what we get from the immunisation of vaccination. Frequent and recurrent infections of the ear, skin or sinus, pneumonia, bronchitis or meningitis, inflammation and infection of internal organs, blood disorders such as low platelets counts or anaemia are some of the most glaring signs of low immunity. In modern times, stress is the primary cause of low levels of immunity.

Millions of Covid-19 patients cured who quarantined. A positive attitude, zest for life and self-confidence were the panacea for their quick recovery. Even many senior and super senior citizens with single or multiple co-morbidities have come back from the hospital with a corona cure. Despite having some co-morbidities, there are several recovery cases for nonagenarians, centenarian Covid-19 patients. Those with co-morbidities like hypertension, diabetes, ischemic heart disease, kidney failure, and a weak low level of self-confidence succumbed to pandemics. Covid-19 patients who got cured also told if there are no symptoms, we need not get tested for coronavirus. It is in tune with my concept that getting an annual blood test and body check-up is unnecessary as long as we feel fit. Self-confidence is the main thing in life. If we do not have faith in the doctor, our illness will not be cured by their prescribed medicines. We should remove the fear in our minds that we have some sickness. You be confident, calm and wait for the disease to vanish. The mind is a powerful tool. More sickness starts in the mind. When I was in the bank's service, our bank reimbursed our annual health check-up after 45. Our bank's doctor was asking me once, "Mr Hegde what is wrong with you when the bank is paying why you are not going for annual medical check-up?" Somehow I was not serious about such medical check-ups because many of my colleagues had health check-ups, and later they became regular tablet takers for one or the other disease. However, now without any annual health check-up, I continue to lead a life without regular medicine.

I recollected my memory when I was a schoolchild. Several doctors were putting RMP (Registered Medical Practitioner) in front of their name on the board in their clinic. Their knowledge and experience in treating patients gave them the confidence to do the medical practice. They had some certificates from some medical colleges of Ayurveda or Unani. Some of them also had mastered the art of administering injections since patients thought injection would cure them fast, and the doctor used to give some glucose injection to satisfy and keep his profession growing. Surprisingly they were so popular in the local area people used to visit them in large numbers. They also charged very nominal fees. The doctor gave some white powder in paper sachets and coloured liquid mixtures in a bottle as medicines to take two or three times a day for three days. The patients had to carry the empty bottle with them. First, the doctor talks friendly while checking the pulse, holding the hand, asking for symptoms, putting the stethoscope on the chest, and asking the patients to show the tongue and eyes. He will also prescribe some restrictions for some items in the regular meal of the patients. Then he assures the patients, "Nothing to worry, the illness will be cured within 3-4 days". Due to the placebo effect, it was such a wonderful experience that most of them got cured. There were no modern facilities like a blood test, or x rays were available in the vicinity. The Villages used to be cut off for 3- 4 months in the rainy season. The faith and confidence of the patients in the doctor were the main factors. The healing process of nature and hand touch therapy were doing wonders rather than the medicines. Further, in the olden days, the doctor and patient relationship had mutual faith. But nowadays, with medico-legal issues increasing, doctors also take precautions before prescribing any treatment.

Our body has a natural healing mechanism for many diseases. Dr. B.M.Hegde says routine illnesses such as sore throat, flu-like infection, common cold and feverish cold come under minor illness syndrome. It cures naturally with simple Indian home remedies like sipping hot water, hot tea, or coffee inhaling steam. Incidentally, I may add here that Dr. B. M. Hegde is a Padma Bhushan Awardee, Cardiologist, Medical Scientist. I am a member of "drbmhegdefan's club" on Facebook, which has more than 500K followers now, and it is growing day by day.[5]

Most medical tests avoidable: An interesting fact has been revealed by a research study on medical check-ups now advertised by the hospitals in Mumbai, which are in tune with the opinion of Dr. B.M.Hegde. It would be prudent to rush for an annual health check-up in a country where every third adult has hypertension, and heart attacks occur a decade earlier than they do in Westerners. But an assessment of 25 health packages offered by eight clinics and hospitals in Mumbai showed that most tests don't have a bearing on an individual's overall health.

Dr. Yash Lokhandawala, the principal author of the study, which appeared in the National Medical Journal of India, said routine check-ups as practised in Urban India are counterproductive as far community health is concerned. Dr. Lokhandawala, an honorary cardiologist, attached to the civic-run Sion Hospital, said that people are most commonly asked to undergo complete blood counts, erythrocyte sedimentation rate, blood group, tests for diabetes and tests for cardiac function.

" There is no rationale for performing tests such as vitamin D, vitamin B12, thyroid stimulating hormone, electrolytes, pulmonary function tests, among others as a part of 'health check-up' for the general population", he said.

A senior doctor said most hospitals offered health checks because they felt it would increase admissions. "They spot elevated levels of some hormones or blood components and advise a hospital stay for a better future to emerge," he said. The study looked at health packages costing between Rs.1650 (for a 'mini' health check-up) to Rs.59500 (a 'deluxe package').

The study concluded that apart from financial and resource burden, many health checks led to over-diagnosis and overtreatment, psychological distress due to false-positive test results, harm from invasive follow-up tests and false reassurance due to false-negative test results.

Dr. Sanjay Nagral, liver surgeon and editor of the Indian Journal of Medical Ethics, said, "Evidence has been around for a long time that health check-ups do not impact health. Leave aside the fact that they don't contribute to picking up diseases. Health checks bring about incidental detection that will lead to a further huge battery of investigations." He further said that he often saw patients who came to him seeking a gall bladder removal operation. "They say a random health check showed that they had gall stones, and they were advised to remove the stones or gall bladder itself". When I told them that non-symptomatic stones should be left alone, they were not convinced. People refuse to accept that asymptomatic stones do not need to be treated. If a fibroid is not troubling a woman, should it be considered a big problem?" he asked.

Dr. Srinath Reddy, who heads the Public Health Foundation of India, said that it is proved that the so-called executive checks are necessarily not beneficial. So what is the best health check-up? It is best to have "opportunistic checks" while visiting the doctor, said doctors. People should get themselves assessed while visiting their doctor.[6]

In conclusion, what we can learn from this research study is that check-ups and tests should be done only when necessary. Regular health check-ups could be on the recommendations of the family doctor. People who maintain good health and are free from diabetes and blood pressure may not require frequent health check-ups. As far I am concerned, I get a blood test once in three to five years.

When we feel confident, we tend to make decisions that are good for our health. We are more likely to take care of ourselves to choose healthier foods and will be active. Confidence can also give us a positive outlook on life, increasing our mental and emotional well-being.

A strong sense of self will help us channel our focused mental energy into our physical health. Suppose if we are looking to exercise more, eat differently, try a new physical activity, or strengthen or stretch our current health targets, in that case, confidence can also be healthy. This helps to develop a healthy lifestyle regardless of age or current physical limitations. One of the first steps to achieving the life changes we want is to believe in ourselves. Believe that we are capable of anything and no one can prove us wrong.

Worry and fear are two substantial contributors to stress, which is a leading cause of insomnia, muscle tension, gastrointestinal problems, headaches, poor eating habits, alcohol or tobacco use, prescription drug usage, and a variety of other physical ailments. Everyone has one or another problem, but we have to come out through positive thinking.

Once our mental energies are dedicated to a physical task, and we can see ourselves as confident at taking on new physical challenges, we can focus on setting ourselves a tangible goal. Because confident people are constantly pushing themselves to achieve new things, and work towards them, and improving their health along the way. However, people with high blood pressure, diabetes, cancer etc., are required to get annual health check-ups and treatment. So also, people with ailments to body organs such as ear, throat, nose (ENT), dental and eyes should have regular check-up and treatment. Further, in case of accidents, we have to get instant medical help invariably as many times surgery may be necessary. Suppose one can do aerobic exercises like walking daily, proving that he is fit concerning heart and lungs. As long as one feels hungry, gets good sleep, and takes healthy food, one's immunity will be intact to fight against diseases. In such cases, an annual health check-up may not be necessary, but it depends on the individual's self-confidence in their health.

Using our present confidence level on our mental and physical abilities, we can become healthier, and therefore, happier. I quote Ironman Triathlon and RAAM racing events where participants build self-confidence to peak level to earn the title.

Ironman Triathlon: An Ironman Triathlon is a series of long-distance races organised by the World Triathlon Corporation. The triathlon includes a 3.86-km swim, a 180.2-km cycle ride, and a 42.2-km marathon run raced in that order without a break, which the participants must complete within 17 hours to win the title "Ironman".[7,8] It is widely considered one of the most challenging one-day ultimate endurance sporting events in the world. Most triathlons involve open water swimming in a river, lake, bay or ocean rather than pool swimming. My nephew, Bhushan Walzade, 33, an executive in an MNC, Bangalore, won the title by completing at Busselton, a coastal town in Western Australia, on December 1, 2019. It is an excellent test of physical endurance and mental strength. Those persons who are committed, focused, passionate and disciplined only could be winners in this event. The person has to face a tough challenge to withstand pain, sustain long training hours, and possess the perseverance to become an Ironman. The mind needs to be conditioned first. I could watch this exciting event live sitting in my home every minute of Bhushan's movements as the organisers had released an app that worked based on GPS tracking.

Another story for self-confidence from Japan: Japanese are known for discipline for time, work, food and fitness as the country has the highest number of centenarians in the world. Hiromu Inada won the Ironman world championship at the age of 85 and held already the title of the world's oldest Ironman. But he does not seem to be stopping anytime soon; World's oldest Ironman is gearing up for the championship's next edition. The enthusiast hopes to continue competing into his 90s. This Japanese athlete began swimming and running and bought a bike at the age of 69. He completed his first triathlon a year later. And with his wife's death soon afterwards, Ironman competitions became an obsession for him. However, the championship of the 2020 edition was cancelled due to the coronavirus pandemic. Inada continues his gruelling training schedule with the hope to return to the event in Hawaii in the coming year. The Ironman wakes up at 4:30 AM and hits the swimming pool by 6 AM. "I hope I can try new things to build my fitness."I hope I can adjust my physical peak to the postponed race. So, I would instead think it was good that it was delayed," he further said. (Credit: Indian Express August 28, 2020).[9]

Race Across America (RAAM): This toughest bicycle race is one of the world's most respected and longest-running ultra-endurance events. RAAM is seen as a pinnacle of athletic achievement in cycling circles and the most beautiful sporting community. There is no other race that combines distance, terrain and weather. No other event that tests a team's spirit from beginning to end. RAAM cyclists have to face desert heat, Cold Mountain passes and unpredictable winds. The race started in 1982, by four individuals from Santa Monica in Pier in Los Angeles to the Empire State Building in New York City. Racer must cycle 4800 km across 12 states of the United States. The team racers have a maximum of 9 days, and the solo racer has 12 days to complete. It is, in principle, a non-stop event from start to finish. Having to ride continuously for days with little or no sleep puts this event in the category of ultra-distance cycling races. The race takes place on open roads, forcing participants to deal with sometimes dangerous traffic conditions. Racer will get hardly 2-3 hours of sleep every day.[10] Why I am quoting these examples is to display how self-confidence builds body fitness consciousness.

Another role model: Usha Soman, the octogenarian, the mother of Milind Soman, super model-actor-Ironman Triathlon titleholder and fitness icon of India, shows that age is only a number. In 2020, Milind posted a motivational video of a son-mother duo doing a rope jumping exercise on the terrace during lockdown due to coronavirus in his social media. When 78, Usha completed a 100-km walk for the Oxfam Trailwalker event in 41 hours against a maximum of 48 hours. When 76, she walked barefoot in the last leg of his son's two-week-long marathon between Ahmedabad and Mumbai, though she started trekking at the age of 60. Age does not make anyone weaker or less fit. She says, "If you think negatively you will not be able do anything new unless you actually try them out. Always keep a positive framework in the mind. Fitness is not to be restricted to body. The mind which drives the body must also be kept fit". Instagram account of Ankita Konwar, her daughter-in-law, reads "In 2019, she chose to go scuba diving in Bali and 2020, she was supposed to go bungee jumping in Zambia (The highest commercial bridge 111 metres jump in the world) to have a thrilling experience but due to coronavirus she had to cancel". Such is the level of self-confidence of Usha Soman.

Natural Doctor No.2. Sleep

Sleep is a prerequisite for our good health. Good sleep makes us feel better, more alert, energetic and better able to concentrate and perform our daily tasks besides reducing the risk of illness. Sleep enhances our ability to remove waste products from the brain, which can harm brain function. Sleep plays a vital role in regulating our circadian rhythm or internal clock. Our circadian rhythm is a 24-hour internal clock running in the background of our brain and cycles between sleepiness and alertness at regular intervals. It is also known as our sleep-wake cycle. The natural cycle of physical, mental, and behavioural changes that the body goes through in a 24-hour cycle. Circadian rhythms are affected mainly by light and darkness. And are controlled by a small area in the middle of the brain. Circadian rhythm is sometimes called the "body's clock." It also helps to regulate metabolism, immune function and inflammation. Sleeping is a basic need like eating, drinking and breathing for good health and well-being throughout our life. Not getting enough sleep alters insulin resistance, which is associated with an increased risk of developing type 2 diabetes, which can be very quickly induced by a single night's total sleep loss. Sleep deprivation also increases the chances of developing chronic diseases like obesity or diabetes, kidney disease, high blood pressure and even Alzheimer's disease.[11]

Old age people require 7 to 8 hours of sleep per night. But rest also depends on genetic make-up. It is important to observe our sleeping hours to determine the right amount of sleep. Some people are happy with just 6 hours of sleep whereas some other require 8 hours. It is the quality of sleep, not the quantity.

Sleep experts suggest the following tips for a night of good sleep: Follow sleep discipline by sticking to a fixed wake-up and bedtime daily routine, which helps regulate our inner body clock. An irregular sleep schedule results in poor sleep quality and duration. Several studies have shown being inactive during the daytime also causes poor sleep. So it is suggested to undertake activities like exercise, walking, jogging, prayers chanting and meditation, or volunteer activities. Sleeping at the wrong time of the day affects the body's natural clock. Our immune system relies on sleep to stay healthy. Staying up late and sleeping in late on weekends can disrupt our body clock's sleep-wake rhythm. Sleep does not recognise the days as working days or holidays. Sleep becomes elusive, especially when anxiety and stress levels are high.

Napping during the day may provide a boost in alertness in performance. If one has trouble falling asleep at night, limit naps for no more than 20 minutes. I quote examples of some of my septuagenarian friends. "A" never takes a nap during the day. He watches his favourite old movies during nap time (2 to 4 PM). One friend, "B", always goes to the public library to read books and newspapers of his choice. "C" takes one hour nap daily. Still, he says he is getting an uninterrupted night's sound sleep. Let us listen to my friend "D", who travels daily to his office in Mumbai on a public bus. 'The moment I sit on the bus, I fall asleep. I can sleep any time anywhere because I go to meditation mode instantaneously. I often passed my destination in sleep and got down only after 2-3 stops when the conductor reminded me. That is because I have no negative thoughts haunting my mind." About me, I take about 20 to 30 minutes nap after lunch, making the room darker. It gives me a refreshed feeling to undertake my routine tasks like browsing the internet, writing, reading and other household chores.

I usually go to bed at 10:30 PM and wake up at 5:30 AM. During the night, I go to the washroom once to empty my bladder, but I do not look at the clock to avoid worrying about the sleep break. Again within 5-10 minutes, I fall asleep. When I was a sexagenarian, I used to work in the office from 10 AM to 5 PM; hence there was no question of napping, but still, I had the same night sleep schedule stated above.

Sleep plays an essential role in our physical health. One of the main functions of sleep is to provide the cells and tissues with an opportunity to recover from the wear and tear of daily life. Primary vital functions of the body such as tissue repair, muscle growth and protein synthesis occur almost exclusively during sleep. Insufficient sleep may cause health problems by altering hormones involved in such processes as metabolism, appetite regulation, and stress response. Sleep plays a housekeeping role that removes toxins in our brain that build up while we are awake. Sleep is the equal partner in the process required to build immunity, strength, endurance and muscle in our body.

Sleep keeps us healthy and functioning well as it lets our body and brain repair, restore and re-energise. If one does not have enough sleep, he might experience side effects like poor memory and focus, weakened immunity and mood swings. Stress and sleep go hand in hand. When we cannot sleep, we worry. And if we worry, we cannot sleep. A good night's sleep blocks the chain reaction of chemicals in the body that cause stress.

Some people say that the mattress and pillows they use do not give comfortable sleep. They go after advertisements of mattress and pillow manufacturing companies who do colossal business. But the bed and pillows have nothing to do with getting good sleep. It is our mind which is free of mental worries, that brings good sleep. Those who do not sleep easily may do the meditation lying in bed by concentrating the mind on observing their breath, inhaling and exhaling to fall asleep quickly.

World Sleep Day: It is an annual event intended to be a celebration of sleep and a call to action on important issues related to sleep, including medicine, education, social aspects and driving. It is organised by the World Sleep Day Committee of the World Sleep Society. It aims to lessen the burden of sleep problems on society through better prevention and management of sleep disorders. World Sleep Day is held the Friday before Spring Vernal Equinox of each year (The spring equinox, or vernal equinox, marks the beginning of the astronomical spring season and nearly equal hours of day and night. The day doesn't fall on the same date each year; instead, it can happen between March 19 and 21 in the Northern Hemisphere; the exact date may change annually but is always held on Friday).

The theme highlights the importance of sleep in a person's life and maintaining his health. A night of good sleep allows better decision making and helps in improving cognitive understanding. The theme also highlights the sound effects of proper sleep, which helps in enhancing the quality of life.[12]

The fundamental mission of the World Sleep Society is to advance sleep health worldwide. World Sleep Society will fulfil this mission by promoting and encouraging education, research and patient care throughout the world, particularly in those parts of the world where the practice of sleep medicine is less developed. World Sleep Society will bridge different sleep societies and cultures, supporting and encouraging the worldwide exchange of clinical information and scientific studies related to sleep medicine. World Sleep Society will seek to promote the development and exchange of information for worldwide and regional standards of practice for sleep medicine.[13]

World Sleep Day 2020 was held on Friday, March 20, with a slogan, 'Better Sleep, Better Life, Better Planet'. The event highlights sleep's important place as a pillar of health, allowing for better decision making and cognitive understanding in even significant issues, such as our planet. This focus is purposefully broad in meaning, surrounding the message to improve the quality of life with healthy sleep. Conversely, when sleep fails, health declines, decreasing quality of life. Sound sleep is an asset to the body particular function.

Natural Doctor No. 3 Sun

Sunlight helps to stimulate the body's production of vitamin D when the skin exposes to the sun's ultraviolet rays. Vitamin D is called the sunshine vitamin. A cholesterol compound in the skin transforms into a precursor of vitamin D. This fat-soluble vitamin regulates calcium and phosphorous absorption and facilitates normal immune system function in the body. It is also necessary for growth and protection against muscle weakness.

One cannot get the right amount of vitamin D from food alone. It is a crucial ingredient for maintaining overall health and well-being. Optimum vitamin "D" level has been a clinical benefit against cancer, cardiovascular diseases, high blood pressure, obesity,type-2 diabetes, cognitive impairment, Parkinson's, fractures and falls, autoimmune disease, influenza, and more.

Sunlight can improve mood. When it is dreary and dark, we feel depressed and lethargic. But when it is a beautifully sunny day, we are happier and more energetic. This mood change is in our imagination. When light enters the eye, it stimulates neurons in the hypothalamus, a part of the brain that influences mood. These nerve impulses travel to the pineal gland, which regulates serotonin, the hormone linked to mood. Contrarily when it is dark, the pineal gland secretes melatonin, a hormone that controls sleep patterns by causing drowsiness. The correlation between sunlight and mood is dependent on the body's natural response mechanism to produce serotonin. This neurotransmitter helps to elevate mood and melatonin, a hormone that promotes sleep.

How vitamin D helps seniors:

Going out in the sun for just 30 minutes per day is enough to reap all the benefits of the sunshine vitamin. It helps prevent the onset of osteomalacia -soft bones and osteoporosis-fragility, the most common bone-related diseases among seniors. They are often caused by inadequate vitamin D levels, which plays a crucial role in calcium absorption. The research studies have shown that increasing vitamin D levels can significantly cut the risk of respiratory tract infections, including influenza. An adequate level of vitamin D intake lowers the risk of diabetes which is associated with physical inactivity.

Studies have also revealed that increased sun exposure may help to protect against certain degenerative brain disorders, including dementia and Alzheimer's disease. When we get older, our skin is less efficient in forming vitamin D, and our diet may also become less varied with lower natural vitamin D content. Hence, the seniors are advised to regularly take up exercises such as walking and brisk walking in open places in the morning hours as the air contains more oxygen during that period. The warmth of the sun can help to overcome musculoskeletal pain and increase joint mobility.

Although there is no cure for osteoporosis, several drugs and medication options are available to prevent and treat osteoporosis. In addition, a diet rich in calcium and vitamin D and a healthy lifestyle can prevent diseases. Osteoporosis is a painful degenerative joint disease that often involves the hip, lower back, neck, and knee, or small joints of the hands. Unfortunately, very few foods contain vitamin D, such as milk, orange juice and some cereals and bread naturally. Cod liver oil is considered for bone health and an excellent source of vitamins.

In osteoporosis, the bones are porous and brittle, whereas, in osteomalacia, the bones are soft. This difference in bone consistency is related to the mineral-to-organic material ratio. Osteoporosis is most often confused with osteoarthritis since often people have both. While osteoarthritis of joints is a degeneration, osteoporosis is the loss of bone mass, which causes fractures, even spontaneously. It is painless until one sustains a fracture. Osteoporosis is due to a deficiency of vitamin D, while minerals like calcium and phosphorus cause osteomalacia.[14,15] I feel that my daily one hour morning brisk walk gives me sufficient vitamin D, as I do not experience any pain related to bones so far.

Natural Doctor No.4. Diet:

"Let food be thy medicine, thy medicine shall be thy food." – Hippocrates, a Greek Physician, the father of Western Medicine (c. 460 – c. 370 BC).

The word diet generally implies the use of specific intake of food for good health or weight management. There are six essential nutrients in a balanced diet: carbohydrates, protein, and fat, energy-yielding, while vitamins, minerals, and water are non-energy nutrients. Calories (Kcl) are used to measure the energy contents in food and beverages. To lose weight, one needs to eat fewer calories than one's body burns each day. Estimation of energy requirement is affected by many factors such as age, gender, body composition, body size, physical activities, basal metabolic rate (BMR) etc. Calories per gram of each type of food: carbohydrates 4 Calories; protein 4 Calories; fat 9 Calories. If we know the number of grams of carbohydrates, protein, and fat in a food, one can calculate its number. When calorie intake equals calorie out, the body maintains the weight; when calories intake is more than calories required, the body gains weight; when calories intake less than calories out, the body loses weight. Generally, physical activities consume 30-50 % energy, basal metabolism 50-60 % and thermic effect of food 10 % (energy expenditure above the basal metabolic rate due to the cost of processing food for use and storage). It is interesting to know that basically, the body will make sure it gets what it needs to function from the food if it does not get it from its lean body muscle mass. Hence proper quantity food groups should be consumed daily to maintain good health.

Dietary habits have to be incorporated into one's lifestyle and adequate exercise to keep the bodyweight within normal limits. As fat contains more than twice the calories per gram compared to protein and carbohydrates, weight-reducing diets should limit the fat intake. Calorie needs for adult women range from 1,600 to 2,400 per day. For men, the estimates range from 2,000 to 3,000 per day. Aim for the low end of the range if we are primarily sedentary (little to no activity). If we are more than moderately active, the high end of the spectrum is more reflective of our needs. However, as we age, our calorie needs decrease. It is recommended to consume food that includes various dishes to accommodate this calorific value.[16] Consuming predominantly plant-based diets reduces the risk of developing obesity, diabetes, cardiovascular diseases, and some forms of cancer. Plant-based or vegan diets comprise vegetables and fruits, wholegrain, pulses, nuts and seeds. Modest amounts of dairy products and farm eggs can also be considered vegetarian foods. Mahatma Gandhi wrote, "He who can take milk should have no objection to taking sterile egg as it never develops into a chick".[17] The diet helps achieve and maintain a healthy weight, reduces blood pressure, and is rich in dietary fibre sources (which protects against colorectal cancer).

Different types of popular dietary plans in the world: [18]

Readers may be wondering why I am quoting so many diet plans. It is to reveal how other diet plans the world over has attracted people to choose their preference.

Mediterranean Diet Plan: The Mediterranean diet is the traditional food that people ate in countries like Italy and Greece back in 1960.

The Atkins Diet Plan: The Atkins diet was initially promoted by the physician Dr Robert C. Atkins, who wrote a best-selling book on diet in 1972. Proponents of this diet claim that one can lose weight while eating as much protein and fat as you want, as long as you avoid foods high in carbohydrates.

South Beach Diet Plan: The South Beach Diet is a lower-carbohydrate diet that emphasises lean meats, unsaturated fats and low-glycaemic-index carbohydrates. Florida-based cardiologist Dr Arthur Agatston created it in the Mid-1990s.

USDA Food Pyramid Diet Plan: A food pyramid represents the optimal number of servings to be eaten each day from each primary food group. The 1992 pyramid introduced by the United States Department of Agriculture (USDA) was called the "Food Guide Pyramid" or "Eating Right Pyramid".

USDA MyPlate Diet Plan: The U.S. Department of Agriculture (USDA), Center for Policy and Promotion, created MyPlate, an easy-to-follow food guide for its citizens, in 2011. The colourful divided plate includes vegetables, fruits, grains, foods high in protein and dairy. It recommends to make half plate of fruits and vegetables and to make half plate of grains whole grains focussing on whole fruits, varieties of vegetables and low-fat or fat-free milk or yoghurt. USDA publishes "The *Dietary Guidelines for Americans*", which is updated every five years. This guideline has one section that gives ten healthy eating tips for people age 65+ to choose healthy meals as they get older. The MyPlate Plan icon shows a personalised food plan for individuals based on their age, sex, height, weight, and physical activity level. The five food groups as per MyPlate are Fruits, Vegetables, Grains, Protein Foods, and Dairy. The 2015-2020 Dietary Guidelines for Americans emphasises the importance of an overall healthy eating pattern with all five groups as crucial building blocks, plus oils.

Hara Hachi Bu Japanese Diet Plan: This diet plan was derived from the Confucian teaching that instructs people to "eat until you are eight parts (out of ten) full", followed by Okinawans in

Japan. They are known to consume about 1800 to 1900 calories per day, which improves life expectancy. About Okinawans, lifestyle details we discuss in the next chapter under Spirit of Living.

ICMR-NIN Diet Plan: The National Institute of Nutrition (NIN) [19] is a century-old India's premier nutrition research institute of the Indian Council of Medical Research (ICMR) under the Ministry of Health and Family Welfare of India, located in Hyderabad. NIN has brought as centenary year 128-page publication "Dietary Guidelines for Indians" be freely downloadable from its website. NIN provides a sample meal plan for a balanced diet which consists of breakfast, lunch, tea and dinner. It also offers the nutritional value of common Indian foods. Details are discussed in the ensuing paragraphs here.

Any diet intervention prescribes the need to eat more whole foods (i.e. as close to their natural form as possible, unprocessed, no boxed or packaged foods). It includes consuming more vegetables, fruits, lean protein (beans, peas and lentils), and healthy fats like fish, avocado, nuts and seeds. Limit white or refined foods like white potatoes, bread, and pasta. With a whole foods diet, not only we are maximising micronutrient intake (vitamins and minerals) but reducing inflammation in the body, which also causes too many chronic diseases.

Our aim should be to minimise our time and money at the doctor. The definition of healthy eating changes according to age. When we grow older, our metabolism slows down, so we need fewer calories than before. Our body also needs certain nutrients in higher quantities. That means it is more important than ever to choose foods that give us with best nutritional value. Nature cure therapy also prescribes a balanced diet well distributed during the day. Thirty per cent should be from fruits and vegetables, avoiding polished grains and five white poisons such as Maida (refined wheat flour), salt, sugar, ghee and excess milk as described in the earlier chapter Nature Cure.

USDA classify the food into five categories:

Fruit Group: Any fruit or 100% fruit juice counts as part of the fruit group. Fruits may be fresh, canned, frozen, dried, whole, cut-up, or pureed.

Vegetable group: Any vegetable or 100% vegetable juice counts as a member of the vegetable group. Vegetables may be raw or cooked; fresh, frozen, canned, dried/dehydrated; whole, cut-up, or mashed.

Grains Group: Any food made from wheat, rice, oats, cornmeal, barley, or another cereal grain is a grain product. Bread, pasta, oatmeal, breakfast cereals, tortillas (soft, thin, flat round wheat or corn flour unleavened bread), and grits (crushed dried corn) are examples of grain products. Other grains divide into two subgroups as whole grains and refined grains).

Dairy Group: All fluid milk products and many foods made from milk are considered part of this food group. Foods made from milk that retain their calcium content are part of the group. Calcium-fortified soymilk (soy beverage) is also part of the Dairy Group. However, foods made from milk with little to no calcium, such as cream cheese, cream, and butter, are not in this group.

Protein Foods Group: All foods made from meat, poultry, seafood, beans and peas, eggs, processed soy products, nuts, and seeds are considered part of the Protein Foods Group.

Classification of foods by National Institute of Nutrition (NIN):

Foods are conventionally grouped as 1. Cereals, millets and pulses 2. Vegetables and fruits 3. Milk and milk products, egg, meat and fish 4. Oils & fats and nuts & oilseeds. However, foods may also be classified according to their functions.

Classification of foods based on function: 1) Energy foods: Carbohydrates and fats like whole grain cereals, millets, vegetable oils, ghee, butter, nuts and oilseeds 2) Bodybuilding foods: Protein-rich foods like pulses, nuts and oilseeds, milk and milk products, meat, fish, poultry 3) Protective foods: Vitamins and minerals like green leafy vegetables, other vegetables and fruits, egg, milk and milk products and flesh foods (dressed meat from cattle, swine, sheep).

Carbohydrates, fats and proteins are macronutrients needed in large amounts. Vitamins and minerals constitute the micronutrients required in small quantities. These nutrients are necessary for physiological and biochemical processes by which the human body acquires, assimilates and utilises food to maintain health and activity. An adequate diet, providing all nutrients, is needed throughout our lives. We obtain the nutrients through a reasonable choice and combination of various foodstuffs from different food groups.

General health issues of the elderly:

Ageing affects almost all the body systems and is associated with several physiological, metabolic and psychological changes. The changes include a decline in physical activity, digestion, metabolism, bone mass and muscle mass. Failing eye-sight and impaired hearing may also occur. Loss of taste and smell perception results in low appetite. Dental problems such as missing teeth, receding gums, mouth sore and jaw pain, atrophic changes in the gastrointestinal tract (GIT), constipation and decreased physical activity could lead to an overall decrease in food intake and poor absorption of nutrients. Inability to prepare food, economic dependency and other psycho-social problems adversely affect the health and nutritional status of the elderly. There is a decline in immune function with advancing age, which leads to decreased resistance to infectious diseases. The increased parathyroid hormone (PTH) secretion in the elderly leads to increased bone turnover, i.e. osteoporosis. The elderly individuals are at risk of osteomalacia, i.e. defective bone mineralisation. It is due to lack of exposure to sunlight and poor diet.

In general, the majority of the health problems among the elderly are nutrition-related. Consumption of nutritious foods rich in micronutrients, including antioxidant vitamins & minerals and fibre and a comfortable level of physical activity would enable the elderly to live active and meaningful healthy lives without burdening society and their family members—resistance to disease declines in the elderly. The common ailments in the elderly are degenerative diseases such as arthritis (joint disorders), osteoporosis, osteomalacia, cataract, diabetes, cardiovascular (stroke, heart diseases) problems, neurological (Parkinson's, Alzheimer's) and psychiatric (dementia, depression, delirium) disorders and cancer. Besides these, the prevalence of respiratory, GIT and urinary tract infections is common among the elderly.

Healthy diet for the elderly:

As people grow older, they become physiologically less active and need fewer calories to maintain weight. The daily intake of oil should not exceed 20 g. The elderly should consume less ghee, butter, *vanaspati* (Hydrogenated and hardened desi vegetable ghee made out of palm or palmolein oil). The coconut oil (now considered healthy) should be minimum. They need protein-rich foods such as pulses, toned milk, egg-white etc. The elderly population is prone to various nutritional deficiencies. Therefore, the elderly need nutrient-rich foods rich in calcium, micro-nutrients and fibre. Apart from cereals and pulses, they need daily at least 200-300 ml of milk and milk products and 400 g of vegetables and fruits to provide fibre, micro-nutrients and antioxidants. The inclusion of these items in the diet improves the quality of the diet and bowel function. The diet needs to be well cooked, soft and less salty and spicy. Small quantities of food should be consumed at more frequent intervals. Adequate water should be consumed to avoid dehydration, hypernatremia (high level of sodium in the blood) and constipation.

A balanced diet and physical activities are the best recipes for health and fitness. Exercise is an integral part of maintaining a healthy life, which you will find in the ensuing chapters. It helps not only to regulate body weight but to reduce the risk of degenerative diseases.

Proper diet and a healthy life go hand in hand, especially for older adults over 65. According to World Health Organization (WHO) reports, most of the diseases older people suffer from a lack of proper diet. For instance, fat in food is linked to cancer of the prostate, colon, and pancreas. Degenerative diseases such as osteoporosis and diabetes are also diet-related, more specifically with micronutrients. We generally find micronutrient deficiency among the elderly due to reduced food intake and lack of variety in their diet.[20]

Foods Rich in Calcium:

Calcium helps our bodies build and maintain healthy bones. It is also known to lower blood pressure. Unfortunately, surveys have shown that as we grow older, we consume less calcium. The body's need for calcium is so essential that it begins to reabsorb it from the bones if you are not getting enough calcium. It makes your bones fragile and brittle, leading to osteoporosis. Foods rich in calcium are mainly dairy products such as milk, yoghurt (curd), cheese, leafy green vegetables and cereals fortified with calcium. The World Health Organization recommends that people above the age of 50 consume 1200 mg of calcium daily. It translates to 4 cups of fortified orange juice, milk, soy or almond milk. Good sources of calcium include such as broccoli, almonds, kiwi fruits, papaya, passionfruit.

Foods Rich in Fibre:

As we get older, our digestive system slows down. The gastrointestinal tract walls thicken, and the contractions are slower and fewer, leading to constipation. Foods rich in fibre promote proper digestion by moving food through the digestive tract. These foods have also reduced the risk of heart disease. Foods rich in fibre include nuts, wholegrain cereal, wholegrain bread and pasta (protein-rich refined flour from durum wheat), brown rice, brown bread, fruits, and vegetables.

Water:

According to a pyramid for older adults created by researchers from Tufts University, drinking eight glasses of water daily was next to physical activity in importance to health. Our body's ability to conserve water decreases as we age, so one doesn't feel thirsty as often. However, our body still needs water. Dehydration causes drowsiness and confusion, among other side effects, so it is essential to stay hydrated. If we take the recommended high fibre diet, we need to drink a lot of water because fibre absorbs plenty of water.

Foods Rich in Iron:

Iron plays a vital role in the body. It produces haemoglobin which carries oxygen in the blood from the lungs to the rest of the body. When you are not consuming enough iron, there's a limited oxygen supply to the body tissues. It results in feeling tired and lethargic. Iron deficiency is known as anaemia. Beans, lentils, cashews, baked potatoes, leafy vegetables, fortified breakfast cereals are some plant sources of iron.

Foods Rich in Vitamin C:

Vitamin C has antioxidant properties which prevent cancer and heart disease. It is also involved in the production of collagen, which gives your skin elasticity and gets rid of dead skin cells giving you healthy skin. It also helps repair bones, teeth and in healing wounds. This essential vitamin can be found in fruits and vegetables. Supplements are also available with approval from your healthcare provider.

Vitamin D

They are covered under sunlight earlier. Simple walking for few minutes regularly outside and consuming milk, yoghurt and vitamin D fortified juices are some of the sources. Naturally, we find vitamin D in eggs and certain fish (salmon and tuna). As vitamin D deficiency also increases chances of falling, seniors should take care.

Foods Rich in Vitamin B12

Vitamin B12 is responsible for maintaining nerve function, production of red blood cells and DNA. As you age, absorbing the vitamin from food is more laborious. It is found in dairy products like milk, meat and poultry products.

Foods Rich in Potassium

Potassium aids in cell function, reduces blood pressure and lowers your chances of kidney stones. It strengthens bones. It is found in fruit and vegetables like bananas, prunes, and potatoes.

Magnesium

Magnesium plays a crucial role in 300 physiological functions. It keeps our heart healthy, our immune system, and our bones strong. As we grow older, our body's ability to absorb magnesium decreases. Some medication for more senior people decreases the absorption of magnesium. It is mainly found in whole grains, nuts, fresh fruit, and vegetables.

Dietary changes seem to affect risk-factor levels throughout life and may even more significant impact older people. Relatively modest reductions in saturated fat and salt intake, which would reduce blood pressure and cholesterol concentrations, could substantially reduce the burden of cardiovascular disease. Increasing consumption of fruit and vegetables by one to two servings daily could cut cardiovascular risk by 30%.

Healthy eating is vital at any age but becomes even more so as we reach old age. As you age, eating a healthy diet can help to improve mental acuteness, boost your energy levels, and increase your resistance to illness. Eating well can also be the key to a positive outlook and staying emotionally balanced. But healthy eating doesn't have to be about dieting and sacrifice. Instead, it should be all about enjoying fresh, tasty food, wholesome ingredients, and eating in the company of family and friends.

No matter our age or previous eating habits, it's never too late to change our diet and improve how we think and feel. Improving our diet now can help you:

Good nutrition can boost immunity, fight illness-causing toxins, keep weight in check, and reduce the risk of heart disease, stroke, high blood pressure, type-2 diabetes, bone loss, and cancer. Along with physical activity, a balanced diet can also contribute to enhanced independence as you age.

People who eat fruit, leafy veggies, and fish and nuts packed with omega-3 fatty acids may improve focus and decrease their risk of Alzheimer's disease. Antioxidant-rich green tea may also enhance memory and sharpen our minds as we age. Wholesome meals can give us more energy and help us look better, resulting in a boost to our mood and self-esteem. It's all connected-when our body feels good. We feel happier inside and out.

Healthy eating is about more than just food:

Eating well as we age is about more than just the quality and variety of our food. It is also about the pleasure of eating, which increases when a meal is shared. Eating with others can be as important as adding vitamins to your diet. A social atmosphere stimulates our mind, makes meals more enjoyable and can help us stick to our healthy eating plan.

Dr. B M Hegde's Healthy Diet Tips: [21]

Dr. Hegde, a cardiologist, professor of medicine, author renowned speaker on good health, says, "Simple rule to follow would be to eat when you feel like eating. Drink when you are thirsty. The rough guide could be about 30 ml/kg.body weight. If one is eating three large meals, the breakfast must be the largest, as the whole day's energy needs should be met. Lunch and dinner must be smaller and the last the smallest of all. One should have at least three or four helpings of fresh fruit in between. Keep the total food intake under control to see that you neither gain nor lose weight if you are normal weight. If one were overweight, the simple formula would be to cut the intake by half and walk daily for one hour to lose around 350 calories daily".

The sign of good health is sleeping well, having a good appetite, good bowel motion, full of enthusiasm to work hard, and keeping the mind filled with positivity and universal compassion. Dr Hegde says, "Ayurveda also recommends you eat well; shit well, sleep well; work well, and if you do not hate anybody, you are a healthy person." Complete nutrition is possible with vegetable food alone. Many people are unaware that vegetable foods have enough protein to maintain an athletic body build. Do you know the strength for the mighty elephant comes only from plant sources? Our legs, stomach, small intestine length, molar teeth, and jaw with its temparo-mandibular joint (the hinge joint between the temporal bone and the lower jaw) are not in line with the lower jaw like meat-eating animals. Our mouth and jaw do not favour eating into animal meat-all tell us that we are built to be vegetarian. Eat what you want to eat in moderation, not worrying about the contents as long you enjoy life. Dr Hegde, a vegetarian, suggests eating locally grown food as our ancestors ate.

Even the meat-eater gets his protein from plants through the animals that they consume. A mixture of vegetables and rice would give one enough proteins. If one combines rice with legumes, it will enhance the protein intake. Phytochemicals are the chemicals found in fruits and vegetables that can neutralise the oxidants produced in our body cells due to metabolism, making the cells age faster. It is the concept of antioxidants. Many studies have authenticated the idea that eating vegetables and fruits does reduce the incidence of many killer diseases like coronary disease, stroke, diabetes, obesity, and the protection is directly proportionate to the daily intake of vegetables and fruits. Tomato eating is very effective in lowering the incidence of prostate cancer due to the lycopene content of the tomatoes. Carotenoids are the ones that give fruits and vegetables their colours. Darker the colour, the higher the carotenoid content that protects against cancer. It also showed a good effect on blood pressure, especially in foods rich in potassium and low in sodium, like bananas, orange and white potato.

Indian vegetarian meal with vegetables, rice and fruits would be the healthiest diet. Wheat could replace rice, but rice is better. Rice holds more dietetic fibre and marginally higher protamine levels, a good part of food protein, although wheat contains a small percentage of higher total protein content per weight. However, the level of protamine is much higher in rice. If one could eat boiled rice, one could get many other vitamins in their natural habitat.

Regular exercise and good nutrition are the keys to keep the bones healthy for a long time. The main culprit in the diet is salt. Since sodium exchanges for calcium in the kidneys, the more salt one eats more calcium one loses from the body. Even when one is young, low salt intake will go a long way in keeping normal bone density longer. High calcium content in diet is another vital part of good health. Highly absorbable calcium is in abundance in dark leafy vegetables and beans. There are calcium-rich vegetable kinds of milk made from soy, rice, almonds, and oats in the West. Exercise is the key to healthy bones. The earlier one starts, the better, but if one has been sedentary for years, exercise at any age quickly tries to help strengthen the bones. Dr. Hegde says, "Your health, therefore, is in your hands only".

My current dietary schedule:

My daily routine starts at 6 AM with one teaspoon of honey and drinking 200 ml water in the morning before going out for walking. I take breakfast between 8 to 8:30 AM with plain *dosa* (somewhat similar to American pancake) rich in carbohydrates, protein and calcium. The side dishes for dosa are chutney powder (spiced lentil powder) and coconut oil; organic sugarcane jaggery with ghee; honey. *Dosa* is a popular south Indian dish made of black gram lentils and rice blended in a wet grinder to make a batter. Then the batter is fermented overnight and spread on a hot Tawa pan. Typically, I take a heavy breakfast with three *dosas* with chutney powder, jaggery and honey. Some days when coconut chutney is made, then it will replace all other condiments. Once a week, other dishes like *idlis* or *upama* or baked spiced beaten rice (*avalakki*) are also prepared. Breakfast will end with herbal tea (*kashaya*). The ground mixture of medicinal herbs boiled in milk and one teaspoon jaggery makes a good flavoured drink. Before age 70, I used to take tea or coffee with sugar, but now I am content with *kashaya*. Occasionally, at 11 AM I take a big glass of buttermilk or lemon juice with jaggery (*Panaka*). During the covid-19 period, I also took immunity boosters like *Chyavanaprash* (made from Indian gooseberry with several herbs).

My lunch between 1 to 2 PM consists of a typical south Indian vegetarian meal of Havyaka Brahmin Cuisine.[22] It includes cereals (rice), pulses (protein), mixed vegetables, *sambar* and *rasam*. Side dishes are *tambuli, hashi* (both are yoghurt based); the difference between *tambuli* and *hashi*(raita) is that in *hashi,* we need to add vegetables like okra tomato. Other side dishes are *sasime* or *appehuli* during mango season. However, invariably meal will end with curd-rice-pickle. All these items are served in a sequence during the meal. During season special items from jackfruit or colocasia roots and leaves are also consumed. Even when I was working full time between 60 to 70 ages, for ten years, I was carrying lunch box with two compartments to office, one with curd rice or lemon rice, the other with two *yelakki* bananas (small size) or one Cavendish or Robusta big banana and three dates. But now at home between 4 -6 PM, there will be a light snack, either three dates or geo-tagged famous one Dharwad *peda* (a product of milk and sugar) and spiced puffed rice or spiced corn flake followed by coffee or tea with jaggery. Dinner would be between 8:30 to 9:00 PM. Dinner would be lean with chapati or rice-*sambar*, vegetables and curd-rice-pickle at the end.

The benefit of curd-rice: Almost every south Indian meal ends with curd-rice with mango or lemon pickle. Curd is a good source of protein, antioxidants and calcium. At the same time, rice is a good source of magnesium and potassium, which helps to reduce stomach cramps and pain. Curd also helps to improve memory, immunity, concentration, and reduce stress. Curd carry good bacteria which help the intestine to process the food better.

After dinner, I invariably take fruits to my liking, mostly banana available throughout the year or any seasonal local fruits like orange, mango, grapes, guava, pomegranate, custard apple etc. As banana has been my favourite fruit since childhood, I describe the health benefit. Banana ensures the rugged gut of the gastrointestinal tract; lowers the blood pressure; keeps the digestive tract healthy; improves bone health; promotes high nutrient absorption; helps in cancer prevention; rich in vitamin B-6; a natural source of potassium. Health benefits of orange: Excellent source of vitamin C; improves the immune system;

prevents skin damage; keeps blood pressure under check; lowers cholesterol controls blood sugar level; reduces the risk of cancer; alkalise the body; good for eye health; safeguard against constipation. One vital thing I would like to share here is that I love my food, not bothering much about fat, sugar, or oils. Finally, at 10:30, I goes to sleep. As far as possible, I try to stick to my daily schedule concerning food. I have not explained the food items recipe discussed here because Google search will give every detail.

Natural Doctor No. 5 Exercise:

Exercise is one of the biggest antidepressants as it keeps a person healthy and in a positive attitude. It should become a daily conscious commitment to the body, just like food. Activities that increase breathing, heart rate and body temperature are good exercises. They are also known as aerobic (cardio) exercise. Aerobic activities use our arm and leg muscles giving our heart and lungs a continuous workout. These exercises increase oxygen consumption to stimulate the metabolism process in the body and strengthen the heart and lungs by making them work hard for several minutes and burn calories. It also improves our endurance. Some examples of good aerobic exercises are: Walking, jogging, running, cycling, swimming, rowing on the machine, stationary bike, treadmill, Zumba (a Latin dance form) etc. Anaerobic exercises involve quick bursts of energy and are performed at maximum effort for a short time, for example, jumping, sprinting, or heavy weight lifting.

As mentioned in the earlier chapter, hobbies-trekking - wellness walk, I made brisk walking as my choice for the daily exercise as I found it is most convenient for me. It is suitable for any age group, particularly for senior citizens. Normal walking is a low-intensity workout that does not elevate our heart rate enough to influence cardiovascular health, unlike brisk walking, jogging, or running. Hence, I chose brisk walking for my daily exercise routine after retirement. My height is 170 cm, and my weight has ranged between 63 and 65 kg for the last 20 years.

In general, walking can help maintain a healthy weight, improve mood, breathing, blood pressure, type 2 diabetes, reduced body fat, and strengthen bones and muscles, diseases related to heart and bones. During exercise, the intensity of actions should ensure a 60-70% increase in heart rate. Inactive people over 50 years are at high risk for chronic diseases like heart disease and diabetes.

One measure to quantify brisk walking is "steps per minute", and about 100 to 120 steps per minute is considered moderate-intensity or brisk walking. Fitness experts typically suggest a 6 km/hour pace on a treadmill to correlate to brisk walking for an average person who does not exercise regularly.

Brisk walking quickens the heartbeat, circulating more blood and oxygen to muscles, all organs, including the brain. Fitness experts suggest that brisk walking for 30 minutes at a moderate speed can help to burn 150 to 200 calories. The speed at which one walks makes all difference.

Researchers from the University of Virginia found that women who did three shorter but fast-paced walks in a week lost five times more belly fat than those who strolled five times a week. High-intensity exercise also helps us lose three times more visceral fat around our organs like liver and kidney linked to heart and diabetes. One should make sure to keep one's spine straight and chin up while walking.

Regular brisk walking can boost memory by slowing down the shrinking of the brain and the faltering mental skills that old age often brings. According to a study done at Appalachian State University in North Carolina, a moderately-paced walk for about 30 to 45 minutes daily can increase the number of immune system cells in one's body and over some time. Walking at least 20 minutes a day could reduce the risk of getting sicker by almost 43 %.

A 2014 study published in the journal of the American Medical Association showed how walking from an early age can help one stay mobile and independent during old age. The sample size included people between the ages of 70 and 89. After 2.5 years, researchers found that the group of adults who exercised regularly was 28 % less likely to have an episode of physical disability. Walking releases endorphins to our system and reverses cortisol levels in our body, helping to curb stress.

Walking speed can also provide a barometer of one's health status. Walking outdoor offers tremendous psychological benefits as one can enjoy the sound of trees rustling and birds chirping and watching for wildlife along the way. Overall walking benefits are decreased anxiety, increased revitalisation, positive engagement and tranquillity.

Regular walking, like most aerobic activities, strengthens the heart and lungs, increases overall fitness. It can improve muscle endurance as well as muscles strength, significantly lower body. Walking also helps to drain excess fluid of lower legs and can help to prevent varicose veins through pumping action of calf muscles. Regular walking is excellent for spinal discs, which receive minerals and vitamins through the pumping action it causes.

Our legs: When age advances, we have to keep our leg muscles very strong. A study from the University of Copenhagen found that both old and young, during two weeks of inactivity, the strength of leg muscles weakened by a third, which is equivalent to 20 to 30 years of age. The whole body pressure is on the legs. The leg is a kind of a pillar for the weight of the human body. 50% of a person's bones and 50% of the muscles are in two legs. The largest and strongest joints and bones of the human body are also in the legs. Strong bones, strong muscles and flexible joints form the "Iron Triangle" that carries the most crucial load of the human body. Both legs have 50% of the human body's nerves, 50% of the blood vessels and 50 % of the blood flowing through them.We do 70 % of the activity and expenditure of energy in one's life through legs.[23]

The calf muscle in our legs is our second heart:

According to Dr Louis Prevosti, MD, the human body is engineered so that when we walk, the calf muscle pumps venous blood back toward our heart. Everyone knows that the heart pumps blood but may not know our body has a second blood pump in our calf muscles. The veins in our calf act like a reservoir for blood when the body does not need circulation at any given time. These reservoir veins are called venous muscle sinuses. When the calf muscle contracts, blood is squeezed out of the veins and pushed up the venous system. These veins have one-way valves which keep the blood flowing in the correct direction toward the heart and also prevent gravity from pulling blood back down your legs.[24]

Walking or running enables our feet to play a significant role in the pumping mechanism of the calves. The foot itself also has its own (smaller) venous reservoir. As you put weight on your foot during the first step, the foot venous reservoir blood is squeezed out and 'primes' the calf reservoir. Then, in the later stages, the calf muscle contracts and pumps the blood up the leg against gravity. The valves keep the blood flowing in the right direction and prevents gravity from pulling the blood right back down.

Our feet: Our feet are made for walking. A quarter of all the body bones are in feet. Each human foot has 26 bones, 33 joints, more than 100 muscles, tendons, ligaments, four arches and kilometres of blood vessels and nerves. Our two feet are not alike, one being larger. Ageing starts from foot only. As a person gets older, the accuracy and speed of transmission between legs and the brain decrease, unlike a young person. Only when the feet are healthy, the heart will also be strong. In addition, the so-called bone fertilising calcium in the bones would sooner or later be lost, making the elderly more prone to fractures. So exercising for our feet should be a lifelong task to strengthen the legs and postpone the process of ageing. Our feet are the mirror of our general health. Conditions such as arthritis, diabetes, nerves and circulatory disorders can show their initial symptoms in the feet. Foot ailments can be our first sign of more serious medical problems. There is no danger of stress under brisk walking as it reduces any aches and pains in all parts of the body. A brisk walk for 30-45 minutes daily improves the enzyme and hormone secretions, as the nerve endings of all the essential organs are in the souls of our feet. The best method of walking: When taking a step, the heel should land first, followed by the ball of the foot and lastly, the toe. Heel-to-toe motion allows body weight distribution over the feet.

Fitness to Happiness: While walking like any other form of exercise, the body releases serotonin, the natural feel-good chemical. There is also the release of endorphins which are happy and feel-good hormones.

Cost-free: Walking does not require any special equipment, and it is free. It saves a lot of money in paying gym fees. It should also be kept in mind that a brisk walk for one person may be a stroll for another. Walking at a snail's pace will not give any result in any benefit of exercise. One thing is sure that those who spend time mostly sitting die faster. Everyone has their speed. What is the difference between strolling, walking, brisk walking, jogging and running? Strolling: Walking at a leisurely pace; walking: Walking at normal speed to make a trip; walking, jogging and running are ways we transport our body from one place to another under our muscle power. Walking, for example, is a low-energy-cost activity, but as we walk faster and faster, the energy expenditure keeps increasing. We breathe heavier until we reach the point where the energy we burn exceeds a particular threshold, and the body's optimisation response kicks in, and we change gears. A walker clocking a speed of 8 km (kilometre /hour) has higher oxygen requirements than a runner at that speed.

The difference that speed makes: The average walking speed is 4 to 5 km/h while brisk walking is within a range of 6 to 8 km/ h; jogging, on the other hand, is a mild form of running, usually at a speed of less than 10 km/h. It is closer to brisk walking but with a hang time. Anything above the average jogging speed is running.

Running, on the other hand, is a sport. It is fast, and not everyone can do it because the impact is more than the other three. Trying to run in the first go could cause an injury to us if someone ran for 15 minutes at a distance of 8 km/h. hour, one could quickly burn 113 calories due to the intensity of the workout. The average person's walking steps varies from 1250 to 1550 per km.

It is fascinating to know what happens to our bodies when we start walking. Here is a minute-by-minute amazing chain reaction taking place in our body by walking.

Minutes 1-5: Our first few steps trigger energy-producing chemicals in our cells to fuel our walk. Our heart rate revs up from about 70 to 100 beats per minute (bpm), boosting blood flow and warming muscles. Any stiffness subsides as joints release lubricating fluid to help us to move more quickly. As we get moving, our body burns 5 calories per minute at rest. Our body needs more fuel and starts pulling from its carbohydrates and fat stores.

Minutes 6-10: Heartbeat increases, and we burn 6 calories a minute as we pick up the place. A slight rise in blood pressure is countered by releasing chemicals that expand blood vessels, bringing more blood and oxygen to working muscles.

Minutes 11-20: Our body temperature keeps rising, and we start to sweat as blood vessels near the skin expand to release heat. As our walk becomes brisker, we will be burning up to 7 calories a minute and breathing harder. Hormones such as epinephrine and glucagon rise to release fuel to the muscles.

Minutes 21-45: Feeling invigorated, we start to relax as our body releases tension, thanks in part to a dose of feel-good chemicals such as endorphins in our brain. As we are more fat, we burn insulin (which helps store fat) drops-excellent news for anyone battling excess weight or diabetes.

Minutes 46-60: Our muscles may feel fatigued as carbohydrates stores are reduced. As we cool down, our heart rate decreases and our breathing slows. We will be burning fewer calories but more than before we started. Our calorie burn will remain elevated for up to one hour.

All this happens without a single conscious thought from us - the human body is fantastic. Mind and body are to be in sync, and one cannot focus only on one. Simple prolonged breathing exercises will help to destress, even in the middle of the day.[25]

Brisk walk for half an hour every day improves one's cardio fitness which helps the heart to pump blood at a faster rate throughout the body. The heart rate must go up by brisk walking to make walking work for one's body. One should become breathless and start sweating; otherwise, it is just leisurely walking. Until that happens, it is futile. Any exercise that pumps fresh air in and out of one's lungs is recommended. Leisure walking would not do much. But brisk walking does the needful. One should decide his duration for fast walking exercise in a day in good surroundings like parks and water bodies which can bring more pleasure.

What is my routine walking exercise?

Post Covid-19 outbreak, I have 90 minutes of outdoor exercise and 30 minutes of indoor workouts. I live in Bengaluru, which is known for its lakes. Bengaluru recorded 262 lakes till 1960. But today the figure has declined to about 81. Out of which, only 34 are recognised as live lakes. Doddabommasandra Lake is also named Kempegowda Sarovara in Vidyaranyapura, which falls in North Bangalore. This lake is spread over 50.31 hectares with a perimeter of 3 kilometres. The lake is fenced with barbed wire but keeping only six pedestrian gates and three vehicle gates. I ride my two-wheeler scooter up to the nearest pedestrian gate, 700 meters from my flat. I will not walk in a group. Even my wife will not join me in brisk walking as the walking speed varies from individual to individual. Before the start of walking I put on my mobile app, which shows duration, total distance, average speed, steps made and calories burned. Once my walking exercise starts, I maintain noble silence, not opening my mouth during the entire length of the non-stop walking period. I breathe only through my nose and closely observe nature, say water, vegetation, birds, butterflies and animals. The walking track is surrounded by forest trees, fruit trees, bushes, creepers.

Because of these multiple benefits, other fitness modules like gyms, cycling, and swimming cannot replace brisk walking for senior citizens. Pre-Covid -19, I used to cover a 3 km distance within 25-30 minutes. Due to brisk walking, my whole body sweats. After the walking, I also undertake some hand stretching and neck exercises sitting on the bench in the park. Neck exercise consists of closing eyes and making the neck rotate clockwise and anti-clockwise ten times each and head back and down 20 times. It keeps neck nerves in good condition.

Further, I also swing holding railing in the park adjacent to the lake. My two arms would lift my whole body in a swinging position, making my legs up and down ten times. Due to these exercises, traction of muscles takes place in every part of the body. While returning home, also I come by scooter. Then I wash my car myself both outside and inside daily. It gives work to all body parts as the work needs stretching, bending, standing and sitting and exercises to legs, hands, neck and muscle. Then I climb the stairs covering two steps at a time to reach my flat, which is on the third floor. These two steps at a time for climbing stairs are also recommended by Dr. Hinohara, who lived for 105 years in Tokyo and led an active life till death. Keeping Dr. Hinohara as my role model, I sparingly use lifts in my apartment. Readers may also wonder why I ride the scooter for such a short distance. As age advances, the ability of the body to balance and correct oneself to slip reduces.

Riding a two-wheeler gives greater self-confidence about body fitness over 60, as balancing the body is more complicated than driving a car. Due to the Covid-19 pandemic lockdown, I changed my brisk walking around the lake to making rounds within our apartment complex. One round makes half a kilometre in our complex. I increased my brisk walking distance to 5 km, which I finish by making ten rounds within 45 - 50 minutes. My walking app also shows an average speed of 6 to 7 km/hr with 6000 to 6300 steps and 200 to 230 calories burned. After the brisk walking, other outdoor activities are neck exercise, body swinging and car washing which take about 40 minutes. Indoor activities consist of deep breathing, prayer, worship and meditation of 30 minutes.

A recent study shows that walking as little as two hours per week can help live longer and reduce the risk of diseases. Six hours of walking per week reduces the risk of cancer and death. Walking activities activate the lymphatic system, eliminates body toxins, fights infection and strengthens immunity.

Good features of walking shoes: Wearing comfortable walking shoes that fit our feet can help prevent injuries such as blisters and calluses. Walking shoes should also be pretty lightweight and have a cushion, providing good shock absorption and flatness as they have to strike with the heel and roll through each step. The shoes should lock around the heel. The upper portion should have mesh to allow better ventilation and lighter weight. The shoes must fit the intricate alignment of bones, muscles, ligaments and tendons in our feet from side-to-side (metatarsals) and lengthwise (longitudinal) arches. As we walk, these springy, flexible arches help distribute our body weight evenly across our feet. The feet with socks should fit adequately in the shoes. Proper fitting and comforts are the main criteria while buying. The flexibility of the shoes is the key to brisk walking. Shoes should be flexible enough to bend with that natural foot motion rather than being rigid and unbending.

For brisk walking, running shoes are the best choice. A person's manner of normal walking (gait) results from the functioning of many, including strength, sensation and coordination in an integrated fashion. Many common problems in the nervous system and musculoskeletal system will show up in how a person walks. Due to regular brisk walking, I do not face any orthopaedic problems like arthritis (sharp pain, stiffness, swelling and redness in the joints in the shoulders, knees, ankles). The human adult skeleton is the internal framework of the body. It is composed of around 206 bones fused. My experience with walking is that you walk alone in silence at your speed. When we walk with others, we cannot keep up our optimal speed.

Benefits of walking:

Walking is the man's best medicine. Walking combined with good sleep and a healthy diet can keep the doctors away altogether. According to American Heart Association, walking is no less effective than running to prevent heart-related disease or stroke. Walking can provide more joint mobility, prevent loss of bone mass and reduce the risk of fractures. Arthritis Foundation recommends regularly walking at least 30 minutes a day to reduce joint pain, stiffness, and inflammation. Walking contributes to better blood circulation within the spinal structure and improves posture and flexibility, which are vital for a healthy spine. Further, walking in nature outside the home also provides vitamin D, which keeps our bones intact.

Walking controls body weight and composition. It reduces the risk of chronic diseases, such as Type 2 diabetes, high blood pressure, heart disease, osteoporosis, arthritis, and certain cancers. It helps to build strong muscles, bones and joints. It improves flexibility, mood, sense of wellbeing and self-esteem.

World Health Organization's Physical Activity Guidelines for older adults aged 65 and above encourages them to engage in 150 minutes or more of moderate-intensity physical activity each week. There is a relationship between inactivity and morbidity, and mortality.

One of the self-help books published in 1946 titled "Getting the Most Out of Life" the author Alan Devoe wrote under the chapter "How to Take a Walk". First, he advises a walk should never have a specific purpose. Rather than having a destination, one should simply immerse oneself in the beauty of the walk itself. Second, one must never take one's worries on the walk. Leave them at home. If they don't, they will become even more deeply rooted in our minds by the end of the walk. We should pay complete attention to the sights, sounds and smells. Study the shape of leaves on the trees. Observe the beauty of the clouds and the fragrance of the flowers. He concludes: "The world after all, is not so unendurable, when a person gets a chance to look at it and smell it and feel its texture and be alone with it. This acquaintance with the world-this renewal of the magical happiness and wonderment which we felt when we were a child-such is the purpose of taking walks."

There is no age limit to start brisk walking. However, depending on an individual level of fitness and health, one should sometimes consult a physician.

As per one press report, walking has also become the top fitness choice of the youth:

According to a new survey in India, walking, jogging and running surpass yoga and gym training as the top choices of most fitness enthusiasts. Zumba is also gaining prominence as a fitness form, especially among women.

Over half of the respondents (53%) confirmed that they have at least five activities included in their fitness regime, with walking (84%), jogging (64%), running (63%), yoga (56%) and gym training emerging as the top choices. The results showed that millennials are increasingly opting towards a healthier lifestyle, with 95 % of respondents indulging in at least one fitness activity, like running, jogging or walking. Walking topped the list for fitness enthusiasts as it is a great way to improve or maintain your overall health. Just 30 minutes every day can increase cardiovascular fitness, strengthen bones, reduce excess body fat and boost muscle power and endurance.

For the study, over 2200 men and women and women between 18-35 years were surveyed. This year's survey revealed an increase in women undertaking self-defence activities, with 45% of respondents including it as part of their fitness regime.

Strength workouts have also gained popularity among women in the last couple of years. More than 50 % of female respondents participated in a marathon, half marathon or a quarter marathon. (IANS, Bangalore Times. The Times of India, April 12, 2019).

Research findings on walking: Neuroscientist Shane O'Mara, Professor of Experimental Brain Research at Trinity College, Dublin, and the University of Dublin, wrote in his book "In Praise of Walking" that brains have been evolved for movement. There is a close connection between walking and cognitive activity. Mobility is one of the defining qualities of animals, including Homo sapiens. The sedentary lifestyle of the present-day generation is unnatural. While the physical benefits like cardiac health, muscle development, and improved digestion are well known, the cognitive gains are less known. He further says that blood flow to the brain increases with walking. Walking is a balm for the body and brain.[26]

Mother Nature offers excellent benefits: A stroll in the fresh air clears our head, relaxes our body and just makes us feel better. Sometimes doctors prescribe Nature prescriptions as a medicine in reducing anxiety, increasing happiness. The nature walks would not replace traditional medicine, but they will provide a supplementary treatment. Nature prescriptions are growing in popularity in countries like Sweden and South Korea. In South Korea, the government is establishing "Healing Forests" for its stressed citizens. Health experts argue that the effects of ageing are confused with loss of fitness, and it is loss of fitness that increases the risk of needing social care. Evidence shows that middle-aged and older people can improve their fitness level to an average person a decade younger by regular exercise. "You don't have to stop having fun when you get old.......you get old when you stop having fun".

Even moderate exercise such as walking, cycling or gardening is known to keep you healthy and moving. Physical activity helps flush out harmful bacteria from the lungs and causes changes in the antibodies that propel them to move faster in identifying and combating disease-causing agents in the body. "Even 20-30 minutes of daily physical activity like yoga or breathing exercise go a long way in improving metabolism and immunity." Relaxation techniques like meditation, prayer, or pranayama will also positively affect the immune system. Deep breathing is one of the quickest ways to de-stress. A long, slow and deep inhale and a long, slow and deep exhale known to immediately shift our mind from the state of stress to calm. One can inhale for 4 seconds, hold for 4 seconds, release for 4 seconds for each breath, and repeat 5-6 times.

I consider exercise can include meditation, yoga, worship, prayer, sports, walking, running or swimming, which ultimately reduce stress. Since my childhood, I have been doing my laundry, even today though we have a washing machine at home. I avoid using a fan or air conditioner, which reduces our body immunity, leading to more diseases. However, this is not possible in cold countries where the whole house or office has to be centralised with an air condition system due to extremities in weather. During the recent covid-19 pandemic when our city was under lockdown and sealed down, my wife and I shared our household work wherein I opted for sweeping and mopping the floor. It increases our self-confidence about our health. Because our mind should always say "I am okay" otherwise diseases will enter our mind.

Exercise regularly and be physically active to maintain ideal body weight Rationale:

It is recommended to carry out at least 45 minutes of moderate-intensity physical activity at least five days a week. This amount of physical activity may reduce the risk of some chronic diseases. One should follow a nutritious eating plan and consume fewer calories. Therefore, it is essential to remember that the bodyweight is affected by the balance of "calories-consumed" and "calories-burned." Those on low-calorie diets for bodyweight reduction should have moderate to vigorous-intensity physical activities at least for 60-90 minutes daily. Physical activity is essential for successful long-term weight management and will depend on current body mass index (BMI) and health condition.[27]

Activity	Calorie/hr	Activity	Calorie/hr
Cleaning/Mopping	210	Shuttle	348
Gardening	300	Table Tennis	245
Watching TV	86	Tennis	392
Cycling		Volleyball	180
15km/hr	360	Dancing	372
Running		Fishing	222
	750	Shopping	204
12km/hr			
	665	Typing	108
10km/hr			
8km/hr	522	Sleeping	57
6km/hr	353	Standing	132
Walking		Sitting	86
4km/hr	160		

(Source: ICMR-National Institute of Nutrition)

*Approx. Energy expenditure for 60 kg reference man. Individuals with higher body weight will be spending more calories than those with lower body weight. Reference woman (50 kg) will be consuming 5% fewer calories.

Calories used:

A 60-kg man will use the number of calories listed doing each activity below. A person who weighs more will burn more calories, and more minors will spend fewer calories.

Energy costs of physical activities

Activity Zones	Examples of Activities	Energy (Calories /min)
1	Sleeping, Resting, Relaxing	1.0
2	Sitting (Light activities); eating, reading, writing, listening, talking	1.5
3	Standing, standing (Light activity); washing face, shaving, combing, watering plants	2.3
4	Walking (Slow), driving, dusting, bathing, dressing, marketing, childcare	2.8
5	Light manual work, sweeping, cleaning utensils, washing clothes, other house chores	3.3
6	Warm-up & recreational activities, walking up/ downstairs, cycling, fetching water	4.8
7	Manual work (moderate pace), loading/unloading, walking with load, harvesting, carpentry, plumbing	5.6
8	The practice of non-competitive sport/ games, cycling (15 km/h), gymnastics, swimming, digging	6.0
9	High intense manual work & sports activities – tournaments, woodcutting, carrying heavy loads, running, jogging	7.8

(Source: ICMR-National Institute of Nutrition)

Forty-five minutes per day of moderate-intensity physical activity provides many health benefits. Even more significant health benefits can be gained through more vigorous exercise or staying active for a longer time.

Walking speed may predict survival in seniors:

Our walking speed can predict dementia, shorter lifespan and depression. Walking is probably an activity we take for granted, but scientists say it could have something to say about the survival of older people. Our walking speed can predict dementia, shorter life span and depression. A large study in the Journal of the American Medical Association finds that walking speed may be a good predictor of the life expectancy of seniors. Slowing down, it seems, may mean the end of nearer.

"This gives us another way to monitor our health and explore ways to age as well as possible," said Dr Stephanie Studenski, a researcher at the University of Pittsburgh and lead study author. However, this does not mean that we should try to change our walking speed, she said. The point of the research is that many systems in our body-cardiovascular, musculoskeletal, and nervous- and others- contribute to how we walk. The health of those systems may be reflected in our natural pace.

Researchers analysed data from nine different studies collectively looking at nearly 35,000 adults aged 65 and older. Participants lived in the community-not in nursing homes or other institutions- at the research and included members of both sexes and various ethnic groups. The multiple studies looked at how fast participants walked over a fixed distance at a usual pace, beginning with standing still. They found that the higher the walking speed, the longer a person is expected to live. It appears to be as good an indicator of longevity as age, sex, chronic conditions, smoking history, blood pressure, body mass index, and hospitalisation history in the last year.

For example, researchers found that for a 70-year-old man, the difference between walking 3ml/hr (miles /hour) was four years of life on average; for a woman, it's six to seven years. A 70-year-old man who walked 2.5 ml/hr would expect to live an average of eight years longer than if he walks at 1 ml/hr for a woman. That difference is about ten years. "If we have a natural walking speed that's pretty brisk, that's a good sign of how we are doing," Studenski said.

The study found that walking speed was the strongest predictor of lifespan in older people who were independent or only had trouble with non-instrumental functions such as shopping, housework and cooking. Walking speed may be less relevant for those who cannot do basic activities such as feeding and dressing independently.

"If we are already having a lot of trouble, gait speed doesn't help as much", she said. Of course, this is all based on probabilities, and it's by no means a death sentence. Some older people stroll and live many more years, just as certain people have high blood cholesterol and never have a heart attack.

One important potential application of this research is helping older people decide whether specific preventive tests are worth their while. Suppose their walking speed suggests that they are expected to live ten more years at age 70, which might be an important factor in making decisions about such tests. Walking speed might one day become as relevant as blood pressure as an indicator of overall health, she said. But, it will take time to see how useful it is to doctors and patients.

Role model for exercise: Mann Kaur, the oldest and the fastest centenarian (born 1916) woman athlete in the country, still makes India proud by winning medals in the World Masters Athletics Championships. In 2019, she won gold medals in Poland in 100 mt, 200 mt sprints, javelin throw and shot put. In her career, Mann Kaur, a resident of Patiala in Punjab, has won 31 international gold medals and over 13 national gold medals. She says, "There is no age limit in trying out something new. You should never think you are too old to start exercise. In 2009, I started running and throwing javelin at the age of 93, motivated by my son Gurdev Singh 70 then. He is my coach and trainer". Her son is also a former Indian field hockey player in the Olympics to win a gold medal. Gurdev Singh says, "Record breaking is my mother's feature. In 2016, at the American Masters Meet she clocked 1.21 minutes in 100 mt. sprint. In 2017, in New Zealand she bettered it to 1.17 minutes".

The lesson on our diet and exercise for fitness and longevity can be learnt from the lifestyle of Ms Mann Kaur. A photograph posted on Twitter and YouTube with the caption "You don't stop running when you get old, you get old when you stop running" is very inspiring which shows Ms Mann Kaur 103-year-old sprint running along with her 80-year-old son on 100-meter track motivates everyone to live life with zest. She also received 'Nari Shakti Puraskar" medal from the President of India in March 2020 for her achievements in athletes. She is healthy without any chronic ailments at 103 with a haemoglobin (HB) count of 13 plus. Mann Kaur said, sharing her secrets of long life, "A good diet and lot of exercise can defy age and help stay fit." Her son said, "She is a strict vegetarian and young at heart". Her routine: She wakes up at 4 AM, bathes, washes clothes, makes tea, and recites prayers until 7 AM. Sometimes she goes to Gurudwara, the place of worship for Sikhs. Other times she prays at home. Then she goes to the track for an hour for sprinting practice. At her age, she is fit, enthusiastic, independent, and world champion. She does housework, including laundry and cleaning. When asked what gives her energy to run, she quickly replies, "It is all because of my healthy diet. Even though I developed some back problems in recent years, it is my good food that keeps me going". Her diet includes two glasses of soya milk, chapatis made from sprouted wheat, fruits and vegetables and two spoons of homegrown wheatgrass juice every day but no fried food. (Credit: Sumit Bhattacharjee, The Hindu, Andhra Pradesh, December 20, 2019).

Yoga, an ancient physical, mental and spiritual practice of Indian origin, is recognised by WHO. The word 'yoga' derives from Sanskrit and means to join or unite, symbolising body and consciousness. International Yoga Day is celebrated annually on June 21 all over the world as per UN resolution. The event aims to raise awareness worldwide of the many benefits of practising yoga for holistic health and wellbeing. In this regard, the WHO has also urged its member states to help their citizens reduce physical inactivity, which is among the top ten leading causes of death worldwide, and a key risk factor for non-communicable diseases, such as cardiovascular diseases, cancer and diabetes.

Natural Doctor No.6. Friends:

One good friend is equal to one good medicine......!
Likewise one good group is equal to one full medical store......!!
-Charlie Chaplin

The sixth prominent doctor is a good friend who stands like a pillar by our side in every trouble. As we get older, our friends can significantly impact our health and well-being, even more than our family sometimes. While family members typically act as caregivers for the elderly to maintain physical health, long-time friends could help maintain mental health by protecting us from loneliness and depression. Even if we have one person who understands us- a friend we feel to whom we can tell anything that's enough to contribute to our feelings of well-being. Such a friend builds self-confidence at times of difficulty and shows us good direction when we get out of track. There are two types of friends-All weather friends and fair-weather friends. The latter are deceitful and bond with us for their advantage. They leave us when we are in difficulty, but the former are genuinely friends indeed. Selfless love, compassion and concern are the basis of true friendship. Social interaction helps to keep our thinking and cognitive skills sharp. A circle of good friends can be considered as an asset and social capital.

After retirement, the social capital can decline due to reduced contact with former work colleagues, the deaths of many friends and family members and loved one's moving away. This loss of social connections can have a direct bearing on mental and physical well-being. Socialising can improve memory and longevity as it reduces stress and isolation.

Japan's Okinawa's 160 islands where we find the highest concentration of centenarians on the globe known for a healthy lifestyle. There are nearly 1000 centenarians for a population of 1384,762 (2018). Here one of the secrets of longevity is that Okinawans spend more time with family, childhood friends and community. They never face loneliness and isolation in their lifetime and enjoy longevity.

International Day of Friendship:

Every year July 30 is celebrated by the United Nations as World Friendship Day and International Day of Friendship to foster a culture of peace through friendship. However, Friendship Day celebrations occur on different dates in different countries. India celebrates Friendship Day on the first Sunday of August to cherish the bond of friendship in our lives. Friendships could be the purest form of human relationships.

One can experience the soothing effect on our brain when we receive a call from a friend of over 50 years. Our memory goes back to childhood days and brings the sweet memories of olden days in schools and colleges. It will have a boosting effect on our lives. I was involved closely in coordinating two alumni meets in 2019.

Alumni Meets of High School and College:

I am putting up my experience of associating in organising Alumni Meets of High School and College because of its health benefits. The bonds of friendship and relations are strengthened through the Alumni network. Recollection of the cherished moments spent in the company of old friends is the essence of Alumni meets. It is also an occasion to give back to our alma mater. During the alumni meets, the high school premises or college campus become a hub of sweet memories, fun and experiences. In alumni meets, one will get an opportunity to meet old friends whom we never met after leaving school or college. Sometimes we are not able to even recollect their names also. One will meet our teachers, and travelling down memory lane is a unique experience. It is also an occasion to meet people of the same age and similar professions. If we have ever wondered where people ended up and what they have done with their lives, this is a chance to find out. If we skip such events, we may never see them in our lifetime. We can also respect our teachers and professors and take their blessings who moulded us by imparting knowledge and character building.

I passed out Secondary School Leaving Certificate (SSLC) in 1964 from Shri Raj Rajeshwari High School Manchikeri, Yellapur taluk, Uttara Kannada district, Karnataka State. Further, I graduated in 1969 from the College of Agriculture, Dharwad, Karnataka State, presently known as the University of Agricultural Sciences, Dharwad.

Class of 1964- SSLC- RR High School- 55ᵗʰYear Reunion-2019:

Organising the Alumni Meet of my high school class of 1964 makes an interesting story. My classmate Shrinivas Pokle who retired from Bhabha Atomic Research Centre (BARC), Tarapur, near Mumbai and settled now at Boisar after retirement, took a keen initiative to collect the whereabouts of our classmates. One may imagine how difficult it is to collect the contact details of 29 students (3 girls and 26 boys) after a long gap of 55 years. Sitting in Boisar, he struggled for two years to get information about our classmates and our teachers. Somehow he succeeded and spoke to me (I had settled in Bangalore after retirement), telling me that he unearthed the details of all 29 classmates and 11 teachers with incredible difficulty. To our dismay, we found that 7 out of 29 classmates are no more. And 8 of 11 teachers have gone to heavenly abode in the last 55 years.

He further proposed holding a preliminary meet on December 18, 2018, to discuss organising alumni meet and felicitation to our teachers. He requested all of us to come to Manchikeri to be present on December 18, 2018, as he will also come from Boisar. But on the scheduled date, we decided to hold a 55ᵗʰ-year Alumni Meet on February 17, 2019, at Manchikeri High School. A budget of INR140000 was also prepared. Accordingly, a fund collection drive also started. On the spot, six students announced that they would give INR10000 each and if need be, they contribute more also so that the event should become a great success. Of course, some of us paid INR15000 later. Later, people contributed ranging from INR3000 to 15000, and fortunately, there was no shortfall.

I led by providing secretarial assistance to Shrinivas Pokle, such as designing invitation cards, printing and dispatching to all friends and teachers. However, Pokle called everybody to ensure their presence. Not only had he gone personally to the homes of our three teachers to invite them. At the last minute, we noticed a small error in the invitation cards after dispatch. Only three of our teachers' names were found to felicitate. The directory contained one Mr M.B.Habbu in the expired list. Just before three days to the event, when I was staying in Sirsi, the nearest commercial town of the district near Manchikeri, my younger brother told me that Mr M.B.Habbu is very much alive. How did I put his name on the expired list? He also said that his daughter is very much in Sirsi, and I may contact her about Mr Habbu's whereabouts. I rushed to her house to collect his address and health conditions. My brother was right. Habbu was at his house in his village near Karwar, the district headquarter of Uttara Kannada district. It seems somebody misled Srinivas Pokle earlier that Habbu is no more.

I acted swiftly by getting printed one colour card, adding Habbu's name, and removing his name from the expired list in the Alumni Directory. With a newly printed invitation card, I drove my car to Karwar, 100 km from Sirsi to Habbu's house. When our Habbu teacher saw me, first he could not recognise me. But when I introduced myself and told him the purpose of my visit, he was overwhelmed with joy to see a student after 55 years.I extended an invitation to him and his wife for February 17, 2019, event at Manchikeri. I also told him that he could hire the vehicle for the cost we would reimburse, but he politely told me he is getting a pension and will come on his own. All teachers had the same opinion that they did not want any travel assistance, but later we gave the money uniformly to every teacher. Though Mr Habbu was moving in his house with a walking stick, he readily accepted our invitation. I took one photograph to include in our alumni directory. One strange thing happened when our teacher Mr Habbu came out to the gate to see me off. He had no walking stick. He was excited so that he forgot the rod to walk. I thanked God to avoid the great embarrassment since he came in the felicitation list instead of the expired one. All the four teachers came with family to receive felicitation on the scheduled date of the function, which turned out to be a gala success. We had named the venue "Sweet Memories Courtyard". It was a rare occasion where septuagenarian students were honouring octogenarian teachers. We all became children on that day. Even we sang the same Morning Prayer as invocation, which we used to sing during our days in high school. Since many of us were meeting for the first time after 55 years, we could not recognise each other. We departed from the school when we were teens with plump faces, but we are now grandmas and grandpas with wrinkled faces and heads with grey hair or baldy, some with protruded belly and gained overweight. While felicitating, our teachers were in tears of joy. We also donated one lakh rupees to the development fund to our alma mater as a token of giving back to the cause.

The whole day event was a memorable one as in the forenoon we shared our life experience and in the afternoon we felicitated our teachers. We hosted the lunch. Besides our teachers, we also felicitated lone surviving octogenarian founder member of the High School and a social worker Mr N.S.Hegde, Kundaragi. We invited present members of the Managing Committee and the entire staff of the High School for lunch. One of the heart touching moments was when our teacher, Madam Ms Prayagibai, 89 while leaving from the function, asked us whether we were incurring any shortfall in our budget if needed. She has brought some money to give us. We were all moved by her kind gesture. Recently I leant she passed away in 2021 due to old age.

Many of my classmates had discontinued further studies took up their family professions like farming and business. However, some took up further studies. One did B.Com, CA and worked for a bank. One joined the Indian Information Service worked for All India Radio. I also did my post-graduation, entered a bank and even a PhD after retirement. Six of our classmates could not attend the event due to either preoccupation or poor health issues. After SSLC, I completed a one-year Pre-University Course (PUC) at Sirsi before joining Agriculture College.

Life is a long journey with so many difficulties, but we should always try to be cheerful. Even after this meet, we are in touch with each other. But many cannot handle present-day social network facilities. But I felt such happy moments rejuvenate our mind, if not our body, because destiny only knows when to leave this world?

Class of 1969- B.Sc(Agri)-College of Agriculture-Golden Jubilee Reunion-2019:

I entered the College of Agriculture, Dharwad, for a four-year B.Sc(Agriculture) course in 1965 and passed out in 1969. After graduation, some studied for Masters, and I was one among them. Of course, after graduation or post-graduation, we chose different professions as per the availability of job opportunities like state Government agriculture department, banks and other organisations. We had not had much contact with each other. However, the case is different for our majority of classmates who worked for the agriculture department. They thought of organising two day alumni meet for the first time at Dharwad, the 39th year of passing in 2008 on 8th and 9th September 2008. Then, most of us had retired as the retirement age for state government was at 58 and banks at 60. I still remember my words which I shared on the stage "Every one of us are fit, hale and healthy that is why we are here for this event after 39 years of graduation. This is nothing but heaven only. Who has seen the real heaven which we imagine right from our birth?" Some 35 families participated in this event. Later, we held such meets almost every year with a strength of 20 to 30 families.

In 2016 itself, a decision was taken to hold Golden Jubilees Celebration on a grand scale. A team was formed with different committees. I volunteered to be the chief editor of the editorial committee responsible for bringing out an Alumni Directory. Our classmates settled in Dharwad did the event management. Our people at Dharwad had collected the data about all classmates. It was revealed that out of 101 graduates, 33 had already passed away. Each of us was requested to contribute INR 8000 each, but later, all people have not contributed uniformly. However, fortunately, sufficient money was collected to hold the two days event successfully. I designed a format to collect the required information for the directory, finalising after due discussion in one of the meetings. The form had separate rows like name of the alumnus, date of birth, qualifications, spouse name, children names, contact address, Whatsapp number, e-mail, retirement date, designation at retirement, institution served, hobbies, personal and professional life achievements, message as a life lesson. One passport size photograph of 1969 and 2019 and two postcard size photographs of the couple and family were also collected. All could not provide their (1969) photographs or family photographs. Besides, a photo gallery contained memorable moments of classmates during their college life or later in their profession or even after retirement.

We also kept separate space for articles both in Kannada and English to be contributed by our batch mates on various subjects like nostalgia, reminiscences, life journey, travel, history of our college and present achievements etc. Finally, duly filled forms along with photographs and articles were collected. Our Dharwad people coordinated these activities and sent them to me in Bangalore, where I am settled. However, there were a lot of gaps in the format. I had to contact several people several times and thanks to modern-day communication facilities. Photographs, many times got through WhatsApp and e-mail. Some of my classmates took the help of their grandchildren to send since they could not use smartphones.

I worked day and night to compile these photographs at proper places. One funny thing happened once. One of my classmates had sent two passport size photographs and one couple of pictures. It is sometimes said children are photocopies of their parents. Since two passport-sized photos looked similar, I put a young-looking picture in the box meant for "then" and an old-looking photograph in the box "now". Then I asked him, "Where is your family photograph; you have sent only couple photo".

Then to my surprise, he said, "I have not sent my photograph of 1969 but photos of us couple and my son". Then I had to keep the then box blank and peel his son's photo to paste in the family box. I had to contact all the 62 classmates to get information to get one or the other information. Thank God I could complete the task well in advance and sent the draft to Dharwad for verification. After this, printing was done in Bangalore and copies were dispatched to Dharwad. The event was to be held on November 21-22, 2019. But the first week of November itself, the directories were sent to Dharwad.

It was arduous to collect personal information because many were neither interested in providing information nor participating in the alumni meet. We were to collect data from 68 existing students, but ultimately we got only from 62 people that too not expecting any money contribution from them. However, we had decided to give a copy to everyone and also our professors.

It is interesting to know how people spend their time in sunset years of life turning in to positive. Some of my classmates are followers of some spiritual Gurujis or Yoga Gurujis. Some have joined religious singing groups (Bhajans) and senior citizens groups in their respective places, allowing them to kill negative feelings in old age. One of our senior alumni has turned in to a priest at ISKON temple to distribute holy water to the devotees to engage body and mind and keep fit. Many of us have taken up organic farming to grow fruits and vegetables. Some are going abroad to stay with their beloved kith and kin once in 2 to 3 years. Whatever it may be, due to Alumni Meets, we are reconnected after a long time as we created one WhatsApp group for those who can operate smartphones and are willing to join. Finally, out of 62 listed in the alumni directory, 37 with family and nine as a single participated in the event. The sweet memories of the alumni meet have added new vigour to our life, contributing to our health, happiness and longevity.

Such events are more entertaining than formal functions. Informal non-business chats with childhood friends take us back to our young age, boost energy and bring happiness.

CHAPTER ELEVEN

The Spirit of Living

Longevity and death are mysteries of life. No one can predict the death of a person. But adopting lifestyle changes, one can delay the onset of morbidity. There has been a shift from communicable to non-communicable diseases. The number of people suffering from non-communicable diseases is growing at the rate of 9.2 % every year. India has the highest number of cardiovascular diseases (CVD) and heart attacks.

Furthermore, hypertension, diabetes and coronary heart diseases occur much earlier, even at 50 years and below, compared to the western population. Other non-communicable diseases are cancer, respiratory diseases, diabetes, arthritis etc. Lack of physical exercise and increased stress levels are responsible for the increased incidence of heart diseases. Of course, in recent years, the Covid-19 pandemic has caused havoc. More than 300 000 people worldwide have succumbed to death during 2019-20, to which vaccine is released to control.

According to U.S. Census Bureau, Life Expectancy was 26 in the year 1800, which rose to 47.3 in 1900 and 78.8 in 2013 against Japan's Life Expectancy of 87.32 for women and 81.25 for men 2018. Japan has the highest proportion of centenarians (who reach the age of 100) and supercentenarians (who reach the age of 110) than any other country in the world. Chronic diseases of older adults are HTN (Hypertension, also known as high blood pressure), leading to severe complications. It increases the risk of stroke, heart disease and death; Chronic Kidney Disease (CKD); Chronic Obstructive Pulmonary Disease (COPD), a common lung disease; Diabetes; Cancer; Arthritis; Dementia and Depression.

Interesting facts about the causes and the number of deaths globally in the last three months of 2020.

Coronavirus 3,14,687 ; Malaria 3,40,584; suicide 3,53,696 ; 3,93,479 road accidents ; HIV 2,40,950 ; alcohol 5,58,471; smoking 8,16,498 ; Cancer 11,67,714. It is observed the major cause of death is cancer.

It is also interesting to note that some of the developed countries have the highest number of centenarians. They also have verified the oldest people in the world.[1, 2]

Top five countries in the world with the number of persons age 100 and above per 10000 people. Japan (4.8), Italy (4.1), US (2.2), China (0.3) and India (0.2).

Blue Zones-Longevity Hotspots of the World:

Scientists generally agree that while genetics determine 20 to 30 % of our lifespan and susceptibility to chronic diseases, our lifestyle has a more significant impact on how long we live. Scientific studies reveal that the capacity of the human body is 90 years. In other words, when India's life expectancy is 68 years (2011 census), one can add extra 22 years to our life to reach 90.

"Blue Zone" is a non-scientific term given to geographic regions home to some of the oldest and healthiest people in the world. It was first in 2004, used by the author Dan Buettner, who was studying areas of the world in which people lead exceptionally long lives. These older people also had grown without health problems like heart disease, obesity, cancer or diabetes.

They call Blue Zones because when Dan Buettner and his colleagues searched these areas, they drew blue circles around them on a map. Dan Buettner, a National Geographic Fellow who worked with National Geographic Society to identify areas in the world where people live to the age of 100 free from chronic diseases, heart diseases, cancer and diabetes. His goal was to understand the lifestyles that protect them against diseases of old age so that others may learn a lesson from them.

He studied five communities in five countries that shared eight crucial common characteristics. Besides, there may be many more unidentified areas in the world that could also be Blue Zones.

1. *Nicoya Peninsula, Costa Rica*: They focus on family and have a unique ability to listen and laugh. Nicoya centenarians frequently visit their neighbours, and they tend to live with families and children and grandchildren who provide support and a sense of purpose. In this region of Central America, residents have the world's lowest rate of middle-age mortality and the second-highest concentration of male centenarians. Their longevity secret lies partly in their strong faith in communities, deep social networks, and regular, low-intensity physical activity habits.

2. *Ikaria, Greece*: This tiny island's long history has been as rocky as its topography. This island in the Aegean Sea had been the target of invasions by Persians, Romans and Turks, forcing its residents to move inland from the coasts. The result: An isolated culture rich in tradition, family values – and longevity. Today, Ikarians are almost entirely free of dementia and some of the chronic diseases that plague Americans; one in three makes it to their 90s. A combination of factors explains it, including geography, culture, diet, lifestyle and outlook. They enjoy solid red wine, late-night domino games and a relaxed pace of life that ignores clocks. Clean air, warm breezes, and rugged terrain draw them outdoors into an active lifestyle. Research links their increased longevity with their traditional Mediterranean diet rich in olive oil, red wine and home-grown vegetables.

3. *Ogliastra, Sardinia, Italy*: Ogliastra is the least populated province of Italy. Due to this reason, it offers nature's beauty and a great variety of beautiful landscapes, ranging from the coast to hills and mountains. Here farmers work hard in the field, drink red wine, eat fruits and vegetables they grow, and are taught to respect their elders.

4. *Seventh-Day Adventists in Loma Linda, California, U.S.*: The place is situated at a distance of an hour drive from Los Angeles.

The Seventh-day Adventist church in this sunny pocket of Southern California was founded in the 1840s. The church flourished through the 20th century – and so did its members who view health as central to their faith. Today, a community of about 9,000 Adventists in the Loma Linda area is the core of America's Blue Zone region. They live a decade longer than the rest of Americans, and much of their longevity can be attributed to vegetarianism and regular exercise. Interestingly, Adventists don't smoke or drink alcohol.

5. Okinawa, *Japan*: Okinawa is 161 small islands situated 800 miles south of Tokyo. It s the ground zero of world longevity. Here people have the longest disability-free life expectancy in the world. No wonder Okinawa attracts tourists from all over the world. For instance, one minor island, Taketomi, has a population of 4,000 but attracts 400,000 overseas visitors annually.

Since Japan has the longest life expectancy, let us see the secret of this exceptional longevity. Though Japan has the world's highest share of centenarians, people in Okinawa live long, even by Japanese standards. Okinawa, also known as the longevity Islands, celebrates a remarkable number of 100th birthdays – the scientists have their theories on how it could happen. What are the Okinawan lifestyle tips? Okinawans are among the longest-living peoples in the world. Okinawans have less cancer, heart disease and dementia than residents in other parts of the world, while Okinawan women live longer than anywhere else on Earth. The Okinawa diet consists of local foods. It emphasises nutrient-rich, high-fibre vegetables and fewer protein sources while discouraging saturated fat, sugar, and processed foods.

Okinawan vegetables tend to grow large. In addition, they are considered safer than produce from mainland Japan due to the higher levels of contamination found there stemming from the Fukushima nuclear disaster. Although some have a particularly bitter taste that you may not be familiar with, Okinawan vegetables offer various health benefits, which make them worth eating.

Many years ago, Okinawa's hot, humid climate and natural disasters such as typhoons and droughts resulted in a high mortality rate. Long before the advent of modern pharmaceuticals, Okinawans had introduced kusuimun (meaning medicinal foods in the Okinawan dialect) into their everyday diet by choosing ingredients according to the season and their physical condition. Even today, the idea of kusuimun is deeply ingrained in people's lives and is believed to be one reason for Okinawan longevity. Considered as critical elements to longevity, the fruits and vegetables grown on the island of Okinawa are increasing in popularity day by day. Many of the Okinawa diet's benefits may be attributed to its rich supply of whole, nutrient-rich, high-antioxidant foods. Essential nutrients are important for the proper function of our body, while antioxidants protect our body against cellular damage. Okinawans primary source of calories is the sweet potato, whole grains, legumes, and fibre-rich vegetables.

The staple foods in a traditional Okinawan diet:

Okinawa diet, in general, is lean and balanced, consisting mainly of fish, seafood, whole grains, vegetables and tofu (soybean curd). The processed Western foods that science links to various health issues are primarily absent from Japanese plates. Japanese food consists of very little refined sugar.

Vegetables (58–60%), Grains (33%), Soyfoods, Meat and seafood (1–2%) Other like (1%). Alcohol, tea, spices are used extensively in Japanese cuisine. What's more, green tea like jasmine tea, hibiscus tea is consumed liberally on this diet, and antioxidant-rich spices like turmeric are common. Black sugar (similar to jaggery in India) has been in Okinawa since the 17th century. The idea of sugar as a healthy food might raise eyebrows, but unrefined black sugar contains minerals like potassium and iron that are filtered out in white sugar. Okinawan food influences other parts of Asia, as the Islands are closer to the Philippines and even Vietnam than Tokyo.

A unique feature of Okinawan food intake is 'hara hachi-bu' – which means 'eat until your belly only 80 per cent full'. Hence, less eating is one of the reasons for good health and longevity in Japan. Keeping busy by engaging in one or the other meaningful work and involving social activities contributes to longevity. Continuing hobbies of their like are also important. They also follow 'Ikigai', a Japanese term for finding purpose in life. In other words, one should enjoy what one is doing throughout one's life to feel contentment and wellbeing, regardless of age. [3]

This healthy approach to eating reflects the country's rate of obesity, which is impressively very low. It hardly needs saying that obesity is now considered a killer, linked to everything from coronary heart disease to diabetes and cancer. It is not only all about diet, but the Japanese healthcare system is also considered one of the world's best. It combines advanced medical knowledge and equipment with an accessible public/private hybrid model that sees the government pay at least 70 per cent of the cost of procedures (more if one is on a low income). The Government has also taken preventative measures to care for its citizens.

Even Japanese children are raised in an environment consistent with enjoying a more extended life expectancy. It is reported that 98 per cent of Japanese children walk or cycle to school. Japan respects the seniors. Respect the Aged Day is a Japanese national public holiday celebrated annually to honour elderly citizens. It is celebrated on the third Monday of September every year. Senior citizens are considered living treasures. It is to express respect for the elders in the community, recognise and thank them for their contributions to society and celebrate their longevity. Many communities throw parties to honour their elders and offer special gifts to bring even more longevity to their lives. Japanese citizens, who become 100 years old in the 12 months before the day, receive commemorative saucer-like silver cups as a token of recognition for being very old on Respect the Aged Day from the Government. When the programme was first introduced in 1963, only 153 individuals were given cups, but in 2014 that number had risen to 29,357.

Japanese people are also more concerned about hygiene, healthy food and fitness. They have a bath culture as natural hot springs are found everywhere. It also relieves stress and improves body skin. They also have a concept of forest bathing, where people spend time in nature for healing and rejuvenating. They have family ties surrounded by loved ones and neighbours. Japanese culture has no word like retirement. They strictly observe the diet, stay active, exercise and continue to work as one gets older. Japan has an excellent public transport system. People prefer to train than owning a car.[4]

Important characteristics of Longevity Hot Spots of Blue Zones:

i) *Moderate regular physical activity*: Quite active life as a routine part of daily life like gardening, climbing stairs etc. but not through intentional exercise at the gym or fitness centre. ii) *Life purpose*: Blue Zone Researchers have found that having a sense of purpose is worth seven years of extra vigorous life expectancy. iii) *Stress reduction*: Developing hobbies, listening to music, walking alone, observing silence, meditation etc. iv) *Eating wisely*: Eating less is something one must practice. Stop eating when your belly is 80% full. v) *Vegetarian diet*: The fruits and vegetables, whole grains, legumes, and nuts should fill your plate. vi) *Engagement in spirituality*: People who live to 100 are part of a spiritual community. vii) *Family life*: Communities in which people live to 100 tend to be very family-centric. They took care of their children, and the children took care of their ageing parents. Older adults are honoured in the family. viii) *Involve in social community life*: Isolation leads to loneliness. Hence, join social groups and volunteer for social work.

Dan Buettner also got the trademark for Blue Zone and created several information messages with catchy captions. Some of them are Blue Zone diet: Live longer from what you eat; Blue Zone kitchen: Ultimate manual for longevity; Blue Zone Recipes; Blue Zone meal planner; Blue Zone Life-4 weeks of Blue Zones longevity programming, stress less, move more, live better.

He also produces Blue Zone®Newsletter which one can freely subscribe.[5]

Role models for longevity:

I am referring to a supercentenarian, a centenarian and a nonagenarian.

His Holiness Dr. Shivakumara Swamiji (April 1, 1907-January 21, 2019)

I had heard earlier about Dr. Shivakumara Swamiji, the pontiff of Siddaganga Mutt (a Hindu Monastery) of Tumkuru, situated 70 km from Bengaluru. After retirement in 2007, when I shifted my residence to Bengaluru, I was 60, and His Holiness Shri Shivakumara Swamiji had just turned a centenarian. He is a monk while I am a family man, but still, I made him my role model for fitness and health. Every year in January, I used to seek his spiritual blessings and give my offerings to Mutt. So if anybody asked me that I am now retired and old, I used to counter by telling them that when my Guru is 100, still hale and healthy, how you can say I am old. However, Shri Shivakumara Swamiji lived a zestful life up to 111 to become a supercentenarian. About one in one thousand centenarians achieve this age. He followed the philosophy of Shri Basaveshwara (Basavanna), a renowned religious and social reformer of the 12[th]century who preached "Work is Worship".

He was initiated into monkhood by his predecessor in 1930 while studying in 12[th]grade. He graduated from Central College, Bengaluru, with a B.A. degree. In those days, India was ruled by the British, and very few had the opportunity to receive higher education like this. He was one of the most revered pontiffs in India for his humanitarian work. Siddaganga Mutt provides free food, shelter and education to nearly 10,000 poor children aged five to sixteen years whose parents are primarily daily wage migratory workers from rural areas. It is open to all religions and castes. Pilgrims and visitors to the Mutt also receive free meals daily.

He assumed the charge as the Head of the Mutt in 1941 when his predecessor left for heavenly abode. His life mission turned into compassion towards humanity. Swamiji followed a gruelling schedule of work, worship, teaching and administration, putting over 18 hours a day seeing the welfare of the children housed at the Mutt. During his youth, he travelled in bullock carts to collect food grains and vegetables to feed the children. Looking at the humanitarian work of the Mutt nowadays, many farmers have been voluntarily offering their first harvest to the Mutt. He worked so hard to nurture the students that he cooked the food for them and served personally on several occasions. Earlier, there was no cooking fuel like gas, electricity or solar energy. So he used to go to nearby forest hills to collect dried logs. Later he cut it into pieces to make it as fuelwood for the kitchen fire. Mass feeding has been going for a century as the fire in the kitchen never puts off as they have to prepare breakfast, lunch, and dinner continuously.

Swamiji believed that education is the only tool that empowers a human being to be free from shackles of blind beliefs, superstition and social evils. Mutt runs 123 educational institutions, including two schools for visually impaired children. One can find children of Hindu, Jain, Christian and Muslim etc., in the hostels. Those students who studied under benevolence are now occupying respectable and high profile positions in Government, private sectors and educational institutions all over the globe.

Life at 109 years: The day begins as early as 3:00 AM. After completing morning chores and taking cold water baths, he performs pooja (worship with some rituals) and finishes by 5:30 AM. He goes through his diary to look for the programs for the day to attend as per the schedule. He never missed his morning newspapers. Then he follows to his office and receives visitors and devotees. He regularly took English and Sanskrit classes for 10th and 12th standard students and attended mass prayer sessions both morning and evening. Finally goes to bed around 11:00 PM the night.

He used to take simple food and avoided items with sourness, spices and fried stuff. Usually, he took one small idli (a baked dish made out of rice and blackgram lentil dal)) with non-spicy curry, a piece of fruit and herbal tea (bevina kashaya-concoction made of grounded neem leaves) as breakfast. His lunch consists of a small ball of ragi (finger millet), a little rice with dal and buttermilk, while his supper consists of two rotis or uppittu without onion or chillies and a piece of fruit.

It is incredible to think from where he got the energy to undertake all these activities. He led a stress-free life with a positive outlook. Seer's cognitive abilities were intact, proved by the fact that he walked without stick (exception while walking on steps), read without spectacle, reviewed the activities of each of the educational institutions and wrote individual cheques by himself for those institutions run by the Mutt even up to the age of 109. The Seer was active both physically and mentally and enjoyed the work. He had a purpose of living to feed, to provide shelter and education to the needy children to make them good citizens of India. The Seer believed that changing from one work to another is a rest and recreation. He kept busy in work related to Mutt's day to day management, children's education and welfare, listening to the problems of devotees, reading newspapers, attending mass prayers etc. He was always on the move within Mutt's premises, visiting the office, student hostels, cattle sheds, community kitchens, dining hall, prayer ground etc. Hence he was popularly known as "Walking God (*Nadedaaduva Devaru*)". The secret of his fitness at this age lies in his minimal eating habits and continuous work with devotion and service to humanity.

He was one of the most revered pontiffs in India. The Seer was awarded the Doctor of Literature by Karnataka University, the prestigious Karnataka Rathna award by the Karnataka Government and Padma Bhushan India's third-highest civilian award for his service to society by the President of India.

At the age of 108, he had jaundice but wholly recovered. At the age of 110, he was diagnosed with pneumonia and gallbladder infection. Every time he was hospitalised for a brief period and recovered fully. Again six months before his last breath, he was hospitalised after suffering from a liver tube infection. Finally, he had a lung infection and was placed under life support. But ultimately, all attempts to revive him failed. He stopped consuming food two days before his death and requested doctors to shift to the Mutt. When final moments arrived, he asked that the children be informed about his demise only after their food. Such was the compassion and love for them.

Dr. Shigeakai Hinohara (October 4, 1911- July 18, 2017):

Dr. Hinohara was a physician, longevity expert and chairman emeritus of St. Lukes International University, Tokyo, who lived for 105 years. He had a passion for medical reform and vigorously championed the annual medical check-up, climbing stairs and enjoying fun in all ages, making Japan the world leader in longevity. Annual health check-ups in Japan are free or highly subsidised. The average life expectancy for Japan in 2019 was 84.55 years. He imposed few solid inviolable health rules like avoiding obesity, taking the stairs two steps at a time, always carrying our packages and luggage etc. After spending his first six decades supporting his family, Dr. Hinohara devoted the remainder of his life mainly to volunteer work.

A few months before his death, Hinohara continued to treat his patients, kept an appointment book with space for five more years and worked up to 18 hours a day. He believed that life is all about contribution, so he had an incredible drive to help people, to wake up early in the morning and do something good for other people. He always had today's goals, tomorrow's and the next five years. He has published around 150 books since his 75[th]birthday, including "Living Long, Living Good", which has sold more than 1.2 million copies.

According to a Japan Times report in 2006, Hinohara led an extraordinary family life being a father of three sons and grandfather of six. He completed 64 years of his marriage. In the last few months of his life in 2017, he was hospitalised, but he refused a feeding tube and was discharged when he was unable to eat. Months later, he died at home due to respiratory failure. He is probably the world's oldest and longest practising physician and educator. His life mission was to share the secrets of living a long and happy life. His prescribed protocol is summarised here.

Energy comes from feeling good-not from eating well or sleeping a lot. One should not get overweight. Those who live long have lighter body mass. Always plan for at least one year. A well-planned life could lead to reduced stress. One need not retire when old. Make sure to keep life busy doing things one likes and contribute to society to get a sense of purpose of living. Dr. Hinohara gave 150 lectures a year, standing up to stay strong. Most of us may not have the qualifications to provide classes, but the vital point is to share knowledge and help others. To keep his legs and heart-healthy, Dr. Hinohara took two steps at a time when climbing stairs. There is no substitute for exercising to maintain physical health. Using a cane, he would exercise by walking 2000 or more steps a day.

The pain to the body is mysterious. The best way to overcome pain is to forget it by having fun, just like a child with toothache forgets pain if he starts playing some game. At Dr. Hinohara's St. Lukes hospital, they offer music therapy, animal therapy and art classes. He believed that hospitals should also cater to the needs of cerebral and spiritual activities. He advised not to be crazy about amassing material possessions. It is a human tragedy. Other species do not do this. When we age, we have to reduce our possessions gradually. Science alone cannot cure diseases. Many illnesses are related to the patient's mental state. He believed that those who are negative and hateful in their thoughts are more likely to get sick than those who possess a kind and peaceful disposition. When the mental state is not relaxed, the immune system does not function effectively, and the person will be less resistant to external attacks. Life is most unpredictable, and we should be prepared to face it boldly. Always keep a role model who can provide a sense of confidence and guidance, especially in challenging times.[6,7]

Dr. Hinohara should be our role model who worked as a volunteer from 65 till his death at 105. When a person is getting older, it is necessary to contribute one's time to benefit society. The joy of helping others is something that money cannot buy.

Mr Gajanan Mahabeshwar Hegde (May 8, 1931- July 14, 2021):

Gajanan was one of the twelve children of his father. He was born to a joint family owning an ancestral farm and a home in Kabnalli village, Sirsi taluk, Uttara Kannada district of Karnataka. His father, after the demise of his first wife, married again. He had four children from his first wife (three sons including Gajanan, the eldest and a daughter) and eight children from his second wife (five daughters and three sons). When Gajanan was 43 years old, his father died, and after a few months, a partition took place between Gajanan's family and his uncle's (father's elder brother) family. Then he became the head of the family and managed the farm and home systematically, which can be revealed by the fact that there was always a cash surplus.

When Gajanan was 52, another partition took place among the six brothers. Gajanan and his two real younger brothers moved to nearby Aalmane village, where the family owned some landed property, and this portion came to their share. Gajanan used to undertake all types of farm work such as planting seedlings of areca nut, coconut and cardamom, suckers of banana, stem cuttings of black pepper, the cash crops of the farm, putting manure, weeding, chopping banana leaves required to serve food in the house, cutting firewood available in the nearby pasture land, plucking banana fruit bunches and cardamom, bringing fodder to cattle etc. All the farm work kept him busy and fit.

Gajanan continued to remain as the head of the family. He looked after the portion of the farm belonging to one of his natural brothers also. In those days, the family followed the paternal system of inheritance where married daughters did not get a share in their parents' property. One of his younger brothers Parameshwar (Prof. P.M.Hegde), had good education up to the university level, and he worked as an English professor in a college in Sirsi. I was also his student, and he mentored me to write this book. But unfortunately, he passed away in 2020 due to old age by natural death in his house at 82. Parameshwar was a scholar, poet, author in Kannada and English literature and a philanthropist used to tell me about the great qualities of Gajanan. It seems there was a good understanding among the brothers about sharing income from the plantation belonging to Parameshwar. Whatever the net surplus generated from the farm belonging to Parameshwar, Gajanan gave 60 per cent of that to him who settled in Sirsi, a nearby town. For instance, if two banana bunches were harvested, Gajanan told his son to go to Sirsi and give one bunch to Parameshwar. Such love, affection, and cordial relationships among brothers are rare in the present nuclear family setup. The next generation is continuing this good relationship even now in their family.

Gajanan's daily routine consisted of early rising at 6:30, breakfast at 8:00, lunch at 1:00, tea at 3:00 and dinner at 8:00 PM. He goes to bed at 10:00 PM. He was very strict about his diet and did not take any food in the middle. Gajanan lived with his wife, son, daughter-in-law and grandchildren. He always tried to live within his means, adopting a simple lifestyle. He used to ride a bicycle even up to the age of 77. His dental health was also good as all his natural teeth were intact. Of course, he had to undergo two surgeries, one for hernia and the other for piles. His regular medicine was only one pill per day for blood pressure.

Though Gajanan had not studied beyond the fifth standard, he imbibed qualities of a good human being adopting a healthy lifestyle of three E's (Eat less, eat right and exercise) and three H's (Hard Work, Humbleness and Honesty). His work culture can be attributed to his excellent health. He did all his household work. He may not be aware of the modern concept of mental health, but he knew the value of a healthy mind for a healthy body. If one wishes to live long and healthy, certainly one has to keep the worries away. A strong sense of purpose, connection to the loved ones, family bond, vegetarian diet and movements within home and farm had contributed to Gajanan's spirit of living. He also had a natural, peaceful death at home in 2021 at the age of 91, within one year of the demise of his loved younger brother Parameshwar.

CHAPTER TWELVE

Professional Experiences and Health

I keep this chapter to emphasize that imbibing ethical values in our profession contributes to good health. The more we try to be upright and honest, our stress level will be minimum. But sincere people struggle hard to survive in this wicked world.

1 Manager on Family Farm:

After completing my masters in agriculture, I was on my family farm for about three years. You may wonder why I did not join for any service soon after my studies. When I joined a professional agriculture college, Dharwad, I never thought of any job prospectus. We had a family farm of about 25 acres, but I was proud to belong to a farmer's family. Ours was a joint family, and the farm's size was petite compared to the number of members. Still, I was toying with the idea of developing an irrigation source to raise diversified crops to maximize yield and income. Accordingly, I strived to create four acres of a coconut plantation on modern lines. Traditionally, we grew rice and vegetables for home consumption and cash crops like areca nut, black pepper, cardamom, banana, etc. Of course, we had some mango trees of the delicious pulp and juicy varieties of mango. We would be under these giant mango trees during childhood, eagerly waiting for the ripened fruits to fall to pick up. We, children, used to fight over who would go in the early morning hours because we would have an extensive collection of fallen fruits during the whole night.

I recollect my early childhood days. I was the third among the nine siblings produced by my parents. In those days, having more children was considered an asset to the family. There were people in our villages who grew children up to 18. Of course, the survival rate of the children was also poor due to many diseases like plague, malaria, cholera, smallpox etc. Many had second marriages after the demise of the first wife, including my grandfather. Due to poor road infrastructure, communication and medical facilities, one could not get treatment within time. We always had 5-6 milking buffaloes, and a similar number of milking cows in our cattle shed. We also owned a bullock cart. Selling milk was unheard of due to poor market facilities. So there was plenty of milk for drinking also to make curd. Milk was converted to buttermilk through churning using a churning pin, then making butter and ghee. Ghee is only stored to exchange within relatives. We used to eat homegrown, seasonal vegetables and local fruits like mango, jackfruit, jaman and many other wild fruits naturally grown in the forest. All those stuff were entirely organic. That may be the reason I sometimes think the secret of longevity of villagers in good old days. Their body immunity for disease organisms was exceptionally very strong. Further, they led a stress-free life.

We had thick forest all around, perennial streams and lakes full of water. Our village falls in the rich biodiversity hot spot of the evergreen tropical forest region. We used to harvest plenty of wild honey during the season. Some experts could climb those old trees to any height and remove the honey. Once, it so happened that we three children went out in search of honey with axe and sickle. Somehow we found the tree is very tall we cannot climb. But we did not leave. We cut the trunk so that the whole tree fell to earth, but it was not a mature honey hive, and we got tiny yield to our dismay. But now I feel sorry for having cut the tree. The coconut palm will take a minimum of 7 years to start yielding and bring income to the family. Suddenly in 1972-73, the prices of areca nut, our cash crop, crashed by 90 per cent. The price which used to prevail in the range of Rs 3500 per quintal crashed to Rs 350. Then I thought, instead of becoming another burden to the family, I should earn independently since my parents also spent a lot of money on my education.

Now, I have to tell you something about my grandfather, who lived up to 94 (The longest survivor among three brothers) without any major diseases. As per the tradition, being eldest, he was the head of the family. These brothers did all the farm work together along with family members for the small landholding. They constructed our Mangalore tiled (mechanized compressed tiles) roof house in 1935, using their labour. While my grandfather handled stone and earthwork, the second brother looked after routine farm work. The third did the carpentry work for the newly constructed house. In those days, dried areca nut leaves were used for roofing the houses in the villages; little well-to-do with handmade tiles; more prosperous with Mangalore tiles. Owning Mangalore tile roof house was a sign of prosperity. My grandfather used to say people from neighbouring villages came to our house just to see our house. Ours was a joint family with some 40 members, and everybody listened to the head of the family. Everyone worked together on the farm. We used to sit cross-legged on the ground in a line to take our breakfast, lunch and dinner, using banana leaves as our plate.

My grandfather was a great disciplinarian. He emphasized education, earning on our hard work, staying true to our words, living within our means. Throughout his life, he woke up before sunrise and undertook multi-tasks. He never tasted conventional leaf tea or coffee. His breakfast consisted of only herbal tea with recipe seeds of coriander, cumin and fenugreek boiled in the milk, adding jaggery (black sugar). He was very strict about his diet. He never took allopathic medicines.

The lifestyle of my grandfather was unique. He moulded my thinking in many ways. Ours is a small village comprising around ten families then. Now maybe 25 after so many divisions in the families due to the collapse of joint family structure including ours. He was industrious as our home was the first to own a radio, a mechanical hand pump, a biogas plant using cattle dung for cooking fuel, a toilet and a car. When I was a child, I observed people visiting our home to see the radio, wondering how a box talks and sings. He also established a paddy processing mill in 1952 using a diesel engine and huller as there was no electricity. He lived by the way he wished to live. He purchased one Dodge 1947 model old car bearing number plate MYE411 for four thousand rupees in 1965 and spent more than forty thousand rupees for its repair. The petrol price was 65 paisa per litre.

Now I recollect one exciting incident in 1966 when my grandpa 69-year old while I was 19. My grandfather was in Belgaum, around 160 km from our village known for old car renovation. After a fortnight or so, myself, our car advisor and our driver went to Belgaum to receive the car back. But to our surprise, it was not fully ready. We all went to Belgaum Sambra aerodrome to spend our leisure time seeing the plane's landing and take-off. My grandfather was much enthralled by the aircraft and its movements. He commented, "My dear grandson! I do not know how long I live and whether I would be able to fly in my lifetime. So let us enquire right now which the nearest airport is and what would be the cost." To our luck, there was one Indian Airline daily Mumbai-Belgaum-Goa-Mumbai route. The flight time was only 25 minutes, the distance was only 100 km, and the ticket cost was 250 rupees. He gave me 1000 rupees to book four tickets for the next day flight. The next day we flew to Dabolim airport Goa, and soon after landing, we took a bus to Karwar, which is about 90 km. We made a night halt at Karwar and travelled to our native place the next day by bus, further 130 km south. Thank God! Later, he agreed to replace the old car with a jeep. Otherwise, we do not know how much more money he would have spent on that old vehicle.

He was a freedom fighter and much respected in the local area. He was also a sarpanch (president) of local Panchayat (a local authority covering several villages) and a member of several government bodies. He was the founder member of two important educational institutions, one for modern education and the other for Sanskrit and Vedic scriptures. Both institutions completed their golden jubilee years and are preparing to celebrate platinum jubilee shortly. My father was also known as a non-controversial gentleman and liked by local people. While my grandfather was busy with his social work and court work related to our land, my father sincerely looked after farm work and dairy. Even up to high school, when I stayed in the village, I used to join him to milk the cows and buffaloes. He also held the post of 'Patel'. Similar to ahead of the village, a link between people and local government. He used to resolve the disputes amicably in the villages.

After deciding to take up some job after three years of my stay on my farm, I applied to many places. In the interview, everybody asked why I was without a job for three years of post-graduation. They were thinking that I was having some problem. That is the reason I could not get an appointment for so long. I had a great challenge to convince them that I was working on my farm. Later, in 1974, I got two options: working as an executive in a private sector erstwhile British company and as an officer in a public sector commercial bank to start my professional career.

2 Rural Development Officer in a Commercial Bank- Syndicate Bank:

However, I preferred the bank as I wanted to have an opportunity to mingle with farmers in the rural area. I (then 27) was posted to Kukanoor village (population around 10000) branch in erstwhile Raichur district (now Koppal district) in Karnataka. The area was a repeatedly drought-prone district. Five members branch had two officers including me, three clerks. The Panchayat (Local Authority over few villages) headquarter Kukanoor had no houses with RCC roof and toilet for rent in those days. Most of the homes had a roof with mud or cudapa stones. Houses with piped water supply were also not available to the village. So we two bachelors of the bank rented house with cudapa stone roof. We had to draw water from an open well using a little neck aluminium pot. First, the rope was to be tied to the neck of the pot, and the next rope was let deep inside the well to fetch water. All of us had to attend the call of nature in the open before sunrise or after sunset. We had to cook ourselves as there were no good eateries or restaurants. Facing such hardships has increased my confidence to face many hurdles in my life. Of course, after six months for administrative reasons, I was transferred to Koppal, but I also serviced the Kukanoor branch for the next six years.

It was excellent advice from my grandfather when I joined the bank. He told "My dear grandson! You are going to occupy a responsible position. Be honest and help the farmers. If you take any favour worth Rupees ten from poor people, you remember you have to pay hundred times more to meet the medical expenses of your wife." I kept up to his words throughout my service. The beauty of life depends on the travel on the path of truth, honesty and contentment. I stayed in one place for six years, considered a pretty long time for bank officers. But I built an excellent relationship with the farmers, which paid dividends in good recovery and expansion of farm credit for the bank.

In 1982, I got an offer to serve in the country's apex development bank. I resigned from Syndicate Bank and joined National Bank for Agriculture and Rural Development (NABARD), an Apex Agriculture Development Bank, for a better future.

3 *NABARD*:

After joining NABARD at 35 and I worked in various centres for different periods. I retired at 60 from this bank as General Manager. My ground-level knowledge helped me for designing projects suitable for credit expansion. I was also involved in the training of bankers working in commercial banks, cooperative banks and regional rural banks. I was also involved in bringing out various publications related to agriculture credit.

Thanks to NABARD, which deputed me to the United Kingdom under British Council Scholarship for three months training on development banking to Strathclyde Business School, Glasgow. The course comprised classroom training and field visits to many places like Lewis and Harris Island in Scotland, Edinburg, London and Cardiff. We also made a five-day visit to France during the training period.

In service for anybody, promotions and transfers are inevitable. Sometimes when we do not get transferred to the place of our choice, we feel depressed. But one should not get disheartened as the case of mine. My last posting was Pune against my wish for Bengaluru, but it turned out to be a boon in disguise. Because of my posting to Pune, a great learning centre in India, I could register for a PhD and completed it at 61, which enabled me to continue working in different roles. Concerning promotion also we need not take it to our heart lest sometimes it will lead to health issues even after retirement.

4. *World Bank Irrigation Project:*

At 60 (2007), I decided to continue working after retirement as long as my health permits much before retirement. In this regard, I had shortlisted two organizations and approached the CEO with a request to utilize my services. I did not put forth any condition about remuneration and perks. While one did not show much interest, the other asked me to join, and he will issue an appointment order as per my convenient date. The World Bank-funded Karnataka Community Based Tank Management (Jala Samvardhane Yojana Sangha-JSYS, an autonomous body Special Purpose Vehicle to rejuvenate nearly 3000 community irrigation tanks in Karnataka). I worked on contract here as an agriculture specialist and social scientist for one and half years.

Here I was reporting to a civil servant, an officer of Indian Administrative Service (IAS) CEO who was five years younger than me. A word of caution is that whoever wants to work after retirement should be humble and learn to respect all from top-level officers to peons. Otherwise, you may not survive. The first thing is to forego our ego and should never compare our earlier positions and status. We should develop a love for our work. People will always look with jealousy for retired people why these older adults come and take away our job. I want to quote one interesting incident. One young colleague of mine used to come to my table and beat the table with his fist and tell in a lighter vein, "Hegde Sir! You tell me why the government has fixed retirement age as 58". The retirement age for state government employees in Karnataka was 58 then. Whenever he raised this question, my reply was, "You see I am in good health, I have a zeal to work and I deliver things to the project more than any young person like you because of my rich experience. Hence project has taken me. In case you still have confusion you ask the CEO who recruited me for the project." Even now, when we meet, he respects me with folded hands and seeks my blessings.

While my contract at JSYS was continuing, I saw one advertisement for the vacancy of Senior Fellow at the National Institute of Rural Development (NIRD), Government of India, and Hyderabad. The position was more than a professor post and with fellowship. I applied and faced the interview in front of a five-member interview committee consisting of very senior officials of the Ministry of Rural Development, Vice-Chancellors and Experts in Rural Development. I was one of the three selected. The prerequisite eligibility for the Senior Fellow was retired status only, doctorate qualification with relevant experience. I was then at 62. Because of my selection at NIRD after one and a half year, I said goodbye to JSYS in 2008. I also hosted a lunch for the entire staff of around 60 people on my last day.

5. Senior Fellow at NIRD:

The sprawling campus in Hyderabad extends over an area of 200 acres. The Institute is considered a think tank of the Ministry of Rural Development, Government of India. The Institute offers training to senior officials of the state and central government and officials of foreign countries sponsored by the Ministry of

External Affairs, Government of India. Invariably there will be six national and two international channel training programmes with world-class infrastructure facilities. The well-laid campus has a magnificent garden, faculty and staff quarters, schools, hospitals, and a bank. There were some twelve centres of different disciplines of rural development headed by highly qualified teaching faculty with research faculties.

I was attached to the Centre for Planning and Monitoring and Evaluation. I was involved in training, action research and consultancy assignments related to agriculture, rural development and skill development. I had to handle classes for both national and international participants. I was a member of the team to monitor the National Agricultural Development Project, a consultancy assignment of the Government of India, Ministry of Agriculture. Later I was made as a Project Director, a country level position for handling two projects, one for job creation for wage employment through skill development the other for self-employment, both for the unemployed rural youth, heading a team of young professionals. I had to undertake travel all over the country. I also authored three books while working at NIRD.

I have to tell you about my stay at the NIRD campus. I stayed in a vast bungalow surrounded by a lawn, flowering bushes and climbers. Fruit trees like mango, guava, sapota, custard apple, Indian gooseberry, tamarind and jaman, etc., were within the compound. When I joined NIRD, I did not shift my house in Bengaluru to Hyderabad. Of course, my wife joined me often. So I had to take different roles to manage my job and home, say, professor, cook, gardener, housemaid etc. Since there were several hostels with an excellent catering facility, I used to take lunch at the hostel, but I always liked to cook breakfast and dinner at home. I was watering the lawn everyday morning. Though there was a separate garden department, it is expected that the occupants maintain their compound. So I also used to do small garden work. I enjoyed my work and stay at NIRD.

Another interesting fact is that I had to undergo compulsory annual health check-ups at the institution's cost. The blood report revealed that the cholesterol is a little higher level. So the doctor suggested having a small dose of regular medicine. I told the doctor that I did not want to take any medication, but I would reduce it within three months. So I did regularly 20-minute swimming and 30-minute brisk walking for three months. Surprisingly the cholesterol level became normal, which continues even today. NIRD contract was for three years. My boss wanted to renew my contract for more time, but I disagreed and returned to Bangalore as I wanted to be with my people.

So, after three and half years, I left Hyderabad in 2012, driving myself to Bengaluru, accompanied by my wife. My temporary household materials were loaded inside the car and also on the carrier. The highway journey of 550 km was finished in seven hours, including one hour of lunch. Before leaving Hyderabad, I had a fixed work opportunity in one of the state government training institutes, which offered less than half the remuneration of what NIRD used to give. But I gladly accepted because money should be secondary after retirement. Family and health should become a priority to lead a peaceful life. Here at NIRD, I reported to very senior IAS officers with mutual respect.

6. Senior Faculty at MGIRED:

In Bengaluru, I had finalized my assignment with Mahatma Gandhi Institute for Rural Energy and Development (MGIRED), an autonomous training institute sponsored jointly by the Karnataka state government and the Ministry of New and Renewal Energy, Government of India. The mandate of the Institute is to promote energy fuels through solar energy, wind energy, bioenergy and hydro energy to mitigate climate change impact on the survival of the earth for a living. Here I joined as a Senior Faculty. I had to organize training programmes for the representatives of Panchayat Raj Institutions and unemployed rural youth for self-employment in the renewal energy sector. I also wrote several articles on solar energy, biogas plants using cattle dung and farm waste in rural areas. Karnataka offers excellent scope for solar and wind power. Here I reported to civil servant officers of the Indian Forest Service (IFS). It is a coincidence that when I was working at MGIRED, one In-charge IFS officer who was my boss just for three months invited me to join him at World Bank-funded Karnataka Watershed Development Project Bengaluru, which he was heading.

Moreover, the work was to my liking hence I accepted his invitation. Now, this boss was ten years younger than me. One should never forget that when age advances, we should be ready to work under our naturally younger bosses. He never treated me as a subordinate but gave me much respect. At 67 in 2014, I resigned from MGIRED and joined the Sujala watershed project, Bangalore.

7 World Bank Assisted Watershed Development Project-Sujala:

A Watershed is simply a geographical area where rainwater collects and drains off into a common outlet such as rivers, tanks or lakes. A Watershed is also known as a drainage basin. The land surface consists of ridges and valleys. The development of watersheds means conservation of soil and moisture by arresting runoff water and control soil erosion. Integrated watershed management aims to create water harvesting structures, soil and moisture conservation, land development, maintenance of water bodies and vegetation involving local communities besides providing livelihood opportunities, micro-enterprises and productivity enhancement, especially in dryland areas as a measure of drought management.

I worked on this project for three years. I voluntarily resigned from the project to undertake the freelance work of my choice. I worked on this project as a documentation specialist, bringing out a quarterly newsletter and other publications. I was also involved in the training of officers and field functionaries in the documentation.

As long as health permits, one has to work to keep our fitness at a higher level. Usually, society looks as retired people are not interested in work, and even if they are given a job, they will not do as much as young people deliver. But this is not correct. Unless you express desire, how anybody will come to know you are interested in work. Nightingale Trust, Bengaluru, an NGO working for the welfare of senior citizens, organizes a job fair every year where senior citizens and prospective employers come face to face. People in large numbers from different professionals appear for walk- in- interviews. These people are old but young at heart without any significant ailments; otherwise, how can they seek a new life for keeping engaged even after retirement. I wanted to apply, but they told me that they would not register people beyond 70. Otherwise, I, too, could have attended. The working body and mind keep the spirit of living at a high level.

After retirement, whatever job I undertook was completed sincerely. I loved my work, the people around me, and my bosses, who were also happy with my work. Why I say, this is because nobody told me they do not want my service. I also thought my body should work and earn something. Whatever I made beyond pension, ten per cent of that I donated every month to charitable organizations in the field of providing education to physically challenged children.

8 Assignment with the FAO:

I got an offer in 2012 at 65 from the Food and Agriculture Organization (FAO of the United Nations) to work as an International Consultant in an agriculture extension project in Sudan. Let me explain how my interest in continuing education helped me get this assignment and how destiny shapes our lives! Thanks to my colleague Dr. K. S. Viswanatham, who motivated me to register for PhD in 2005 when I was 58, while in service at NABARD. He used to get overseas assignments one after another for many years. He had been working with United Nations Development Programme (UNDP) abroad for a long time had settled in Hyderabad. He asked for my CV in 2011 when I was with NIRD to submit to the Food and Agriculture Organization (FAO), Sudan. The authorities at Sudan had asked him to forward three names for one vacancy of International Extension Consultant. He frankly told me that he kept me at the second place since the prescribed qualification and experience of the person at first place matches more to the vacancy. However, he was hopeful about my selection, so he insisted on getting yellow fever injection required to get a visa for many African countries before leaving Hyderabad, which I complied faithfully.

I got the offer from the FAO through email in 2012. After my acceptance and signing Terms of Reference (TOR), the FAO sent return air tickets from Bengaluru to Khartoum, the capital of Sudan. Of course, I was a member of the team headed by Dr. Viswanatham. The team consisted of 3 experts, one each of Irrigation (Indian), Geology (Italian) and Agriculture Extension (Myself). The team visited Sudan twice for a one-month duration for monitoring the project. This overseas assignment was very risky as Sudan was under civil war. Most of the international organizations were distributing food, medicare and medicines to the war-affected poor people. The work in Sudan was callous. The scorching sun outside and managing vegetarian food were significant challenges. Fortunately, both of us me and Dr. Viswanatham, were vegetarians. We carried with us many packed MTR and Everest brand food items from India. The accommodation provided to us had a self-contained kitchen. So I became the main chef also. We used to finish our dinner with rice and MTR chutney powder, yoghurt, followed by fruits.

While on our trip outside Khartoum, we carried rice with us, which we were giving to the cook at the hotel we stayed. On travel, we always used to take bread and banana in our bag so that we were not starved if lunch was not available. The local officials arranged food, but we were not sure about its vegetarian purity. Whenever we visited villages, local officials set food in a big round plate where dishes are placed to serve. Everyone squatted on the ground around the big round plate and ate together, taking dishes from the vessel. I was told camel meat is a delicacy in Sudan. Donkeys are used as a means of transport for people, luggage and fetching water from 4-5 km in rural areas. I could see a milkman coming on the donkey along with milk cans and knocking on the door without alighting and delivering the milk to an individual house and going to the next place. During each one month visit, it was 15 days of travel to the field and 15 days of report preparation at the hotel using our laptop as we had to submit the report before our return to India. Most of the days, I used to sleep at 12 night and get up at 5 AM. It shows that five hours of undisturbed sleep is enough for a healthy human body. As per my oath of donating for charity, I gave ten per cent of my consultation fees received from the FAO to charitable organizations.

So, I worked for ten years as a full-time employee after retirement up to 70, in different professions not related to banking where I had 34 years' experience before. I feel this was possible due to my zeal to continue learning and interest in work. Even now, I undertake freelance work like delivering radio talk, Kannada translation for agriculture subjects, writing scripts for documentaries in the agriculture field, contributing articles to journals and periodicals etc. My fitness consciousness keeps me busy as I try to maintain discipline in food, sleep, exercise and work to keep away from the doctor. Adding healthy years after retirement means making life joyful and worth living years after years till we become frail. I feel retirement and age do not affect anybody for doing good work.

Epilogue

Enthusiasm and cheerfulness for work is good health. A recent study in India on the aged reveals that around seventy-five per cent of those sixty and above suffer from one or the other chronic diseases like hypertension, heart disease, diabetes, lung diseases, and cancer. Twenty-seven per cent of the elderly have multimorbidities. Around forty per cent have one or the other disability, and twenty per cent have issues related to mental health. When such is the situation maintaining good health should be the priority in the life of seniors by adopting a holistic approach

Material wealth in the form of fat bank balance, properties, luxury cars, expensive clothes, gold etc., of any quantity cannot bring health and happiness. After retirement, we should stop craving more wealth and material pleasures. The challenge of ageing is unique and very personal to an individual. Similarly, there is no uniform fitness formula applicable to everyone as a fingerprint does not match with anyone another person on the earth. The common saying "We are old as we feel" is the truth. When one aspires to have longevity, he has to be in good health. Hence "Fitness First" should be the goal after retirement. Fitness means not only physical but also mental, spiritual and psychological because all these factors together constitute for health and happiness of any individual.

It is a proven fact that only twenty to thirty per cent of life expectancy is genetic. In contrast, seventy to eighty per cent of the variation is due to attitude, behaviour and environment. Thus the vast majority of factors could be lifestyle modification. Whatever wealth one has, if one does not have contentment in life, one cannot enjoy health and happiness. Even if someone is suffering from any disease, we should accept the reality and live with it gracefully.

One should always try to be independent and engaged, which are essential elements that enable us to manage the transition of ageing successfully. I consider independence means my ability to remain healthy by taking preventive care, health interventions, new technologies, opportunities for lifelong learning. I manage social networks, undertaking activities of daily living like kitchen work, bringing groceries, dusting, sweeping, washing dishes, doing laundry, preparing meals, cleaning bathrooms, taking baths, managing clothes, reading etc. I always try to get engaged in some social activities of the community with a sense of purpose. Adding meaning to life and work is adding healthy years to life. Another important thing is when we age, we have to imbibe the attitude of 'I respect my body"; "I live for myself","I love my food"; I love to live independent to my last breath".

Happiness and health do not come from medicine but come from peace of mind, heart, and soul. Health is not all mathematics but biology, psychology and social development. Birth and death in one's life are mysteries that are not in one's hands. Each of us generally has to pass through life stages in different ways, say childhood, student, adulthood, marriage, parenting, career, retirement, old age and ultimately death. Retirement is not resignation from life. With the present context of advancement in medical sciences, medical facilities available and adopting a healthy lifestyle, one can expect to live long as destined. Still, no one can avoid old age as it is a natural biological process.

Longevity mainly depends on regular exercise, life purpose, vegetarian diet, spirituality, family life, and social community work. I suggest that continuous learning provides numerous benefits for older persons. It gives a challenge to mind and body, keeping the brain sharp.

Developing hobbies and social contacts after retirement is a great stress buster. Undertaking philanthropic activities, including organ donation, is good for health. I am a body donor for research to a medical institute. Anger, hatred, ego and pride have emerged as prime causes for stress resulting in illness. Hence we aim to leave them behind and keep our minds calm.I firmly believe that people who help others have healthier and happy lives. We should develop compassion for fellow human beings.

We should spend more time in the company of children, family and friends. However, when we deal with our children, there can be conflicts due to the generation gap. But without many arguments, we have to accept the reality and better be tolerant to maintain harmony. It is good for us that our kids feel that they have the moral responsibility of taking care of us in our old age. Annual family get together is also crucial for the siblings who have settled in different places for better livelihoods over the years. Our six brothers organize this event in our native place every year, inviting relatives and local friends. When we meet with our spouses and children, there will be a feeling of strength and unity. We carry the memories of the current year and look forward to next year event with more fun and entertainment.

Among so many things available under a holistic approach to maintaining good health, I consider keeping six preventive medicine natural doctors always with me. They are Self-confidence, sleep, sun, diet, exercise and friends. These natural doctors can have a massive impact on our health without any financial burden. These things are also complementary to any medical system, say western medicine, homoeopathy or Ayurveda etc. Sometimes they act as self-healing mechanisms in the body both physically and psychologically. They strengthen our immune system in the body and reduce the risk of chronic diseases.

Age length, which is not in our hands, is immaterial, but the quality of healthy living is essential. We aim to keep ourselves cheerful and happy till the last breath. Though I have been living without regular medicine after retirement, I do not know when destiny will take me away from this world. I penned my life experience to share with the readers. I continue to pray as per the Vedic scripture "*Anaayaasena maranam vina dainyena jeevanam*" (Give me a death without pain and grant me a life where I am not dependent on anyone).

Acknowledgement –the References

Chapter1 Introduction

1. http://www.brinkzone.com/articles/successful-aging-its-your-choice/
2. https://www.verywell.com/what-is-biological-age-2223375
3. WahlinA., MacDonald S.W., deFrias C.M., Nilsson L.G., Dixon R.A. "How do health and biological age influence chronological age and sex differences in cognitive aging: moderating, mediating, or both?" *Psychol Aging.* 2006 Jun; 21(2):318-32.
4. https://www.agingcare.com/articles/chronological-age-versus-biological-age-184345.htm by Ashley Huntsberry- lett
5. World Population Ageing Report, World Population Prospects: the 2017 Revision,DESA United Nations Programme on Ageing

Chapter 2 History of retirement

1. https://www.ssa.gov/history/ottob.html
2. http://www.seattletimes.com/nation-world/a-brief-history-of-retirement-its-a-modern-idea/ *SARAH LASKOW*
3. https://www.adb.org/sites/default/files/publication/28601/ind-pension-reform.pdf
4. https://www.crisil.com/private-sector-pension-coverage/report/crisil-insight-time-to-build-pension-net-for-millions.pdf

Chapter 3 Research Studies -Healthy Ageing

1. https://www.brainyquote.com/quotes/mahatma_gandhi_105593
2. Lee P-L. Depressive Symptoms Negate the Beneficial Effects of Physical Activity on Mortality Risk.The International Journal of Aging and Human Development. 2013; 76(2):165-179. doi:10.2190/AG.76.2.d

3. Times of India Jan 9, 2017, Helping others to help you live longer
4. Times of India Apr 7, 2018 - Older grow as many new brain cells as young
5. https://blogs.scientificamerican.com/observations/loneliness-is-harmful-to-our-nations-health/
6. Times of India Sep 23, 2017-Doing household chores is as good as going to gym
7. Aimee Swartz. American Journal of Public Health Vol.98 No.7, July 2008,(1161-1166) https://www.ncbi.nlm.nih.gov/pmc/articles/PMC2424092/pdf/0981163.pdf
8. N.Engl.J.Med 70.389(2018)0 Why companies recruit people over 50
9. Muthender Velishala http://www.spekingtree.in/blog-to 70-to-79

Chapter 4 Lifelong Learning for Longevity

1. https://www.judsonsmartliving.org/blog/lifelong-learning-as-we-age-benefits-both- mind-and-body/
2. Sandra von Doetinchem, asa(American Society on Aging), Lifelong Learning: Do You Know It When You See It? https://www.asaging.org/blog/lifelong-learning-do-you-know-it-when-you-see-it
3. ttps://briacommunities.ca/blogs/benefits-of-lifelong-learning-for-seniors/
4. Miya Narushima, Jian Liu, and Naomi Diestelkamp , Ageing and Society Cambridge University Press Ageing Soc. 2018 Apr; 38(4): 651–675.Published online 2016 Nov 21. doi: 10.1017/S0144686X16001136 https://www.ncbi.nlm.nih.gov/pmc/articles/PMC5848758/
5. Nancy Merz Nordstrom, Med, Lifelong Learning- Encourage Elders to Exercise Mind, Body, and Spirit Aging Well Vol. 3 No. 2 P. 27 https://www.todaysgeriatricmedicine.com/archive/

050310p27.shtml
6. Lifelong Learning: Good for seniors' Minds & Bodies by Brad Breeding| May 28, 2018
https://www.mylifesite.net/blog/post/lifelong-learning-good-seniors-minds-bodies/
7. *http://prasannacounsellingcentre.com/*

Chapter 5 Developing Hobbies and Social Contacts

1. www.ypsbengaluru.com
2. https://www.bbc.com/news/science-environment-30799436
3. https://phys.org/news/2013-10-alpine-swift-aloft-days.html
4. https://wingthreads.com/oriental-pratincole-update-11/
5. https://wingthreads.com/in-search-of-sep/

Chapter 6 Organ and Body Donation

1. https://www.aiims.edu/en/national-eye-bank.html
2. https://www.ebai.org
3. Nallusamy S, Shyamalapriya, Balaji, Ranjan, Yogendran. Organ donation – Current Indian scenario. J Pract Cardiovasc Sci 2018; 4:177-9 www.j-pcs.org
4. http://www.transplant-observatory.org
5. https://dghs.gov.in/
6. Sunil Shroff Indian J Urol. 2009 Jul-Sep; 25(3): 348–355.doi: 10.4103/0970-1591.56203
7. https://www.organdonation.nhs.uk

Chapter 7 Philanthropic Activities and health

1. https://www.learningtogive.org/resources/philanthropy
2. https://www.forbes.com/sites/willyakowicz/2020/12/29/the-top-10-philanthropic-gifts-of-2019/#db13fa679466
3. https://yourstory.com/2019/08/top-philanthropist-businessmen-charity-donation-billionaires-

india?utm_pageloadtype=scroll
4. http://www.oecd.org/development/philanthropy-centre/ researchprojects/OECD_India_Private_Giving_2019.pdf
5. https://www.unlimitedloveinstitute.org/
6. https://www.stonybrook.edu/commcms/bioethics/_pdf/ goodtobegood.pdf
7. https://www.purdueglobal.edu/blog/social-behavioral-sciences/helping-those-in-need/
8. https://greatergood.berkeley.edu/article/item/ 5_ways_giving_is_good_for_you
9. https://www.canadahelps.org/en/giving-life/featured-series/ hinduism-and-charitable-giving/
10. https://cause4.co.uk/blog/importance-charity-different-religions
11. https://www.kindluxury.com/2018/10/17/one-thing-all-religions-have-in-common-charity/
12. https://hds.harvard.edu/news/2013/12/13/why-give-religious-roots-charity#

Chapter 8 Experience with Nature Cure

1. https://www.ayush.gov.in/
2. https://www.ncbi.nlm.nih.gov/pmc/articles/PMC516460/

Chapter 9 A Student of Vipassna Meditation

1. www.vridhamma.org
2. www.globalpagoda.org

Chapter 10 Possessing Natural Doctors

1. Facts About Healthy Aging | NCOAwww.ncoa.org › resources-for-reporters › get-the- facts
2. Paul Kalanithi, "When Breath Becomes Air", Random House Publishing Group (2016)

3. Atul Gawande, "Being Mortal , Medicine and What Matters in the End" Metropolitan Books Henry Hott and Company (2014)

4. https://medium.com/@sockapalaniappan/the-sky-gets-dark-slowly-146842d772dc

5. http://bmhegde.com/hegde/news.php

6. http://timesofindia.indiatimes.com/articleshow/54385881.cms utm_source=contentofinterest & utm_medium=text & utm_campaign=cppst

7. https://www.ironman.com/

8. https://www.ncbi.nlm.nih.gov/pmc/articles/PMC3582317/

9. https://indianexpress.com/article/lifestyle/fitness/hiromu-inada-world-oldest-ironman- 87-fitness-training- 6573241/

10. https://www.raceacrossamerica.org/

11. http://healthysleep.med.harvard.edu/need-sleep/whats-in-it-for-you/health

12. https://worldsleepday.org/

13. https://worldsleepsociety.org/about/

14. https://www.healthline.com/health/food-nutrition/benefits-vitamin-d#boosts-weight-loss

15. https://www.completecare.ca/blog/benefits-of-sunlight-seniors/

16. https://www.eatright.org/food/nutrition/dietary-guidelines-and-myplate/how-many-calories-do-adults-need

17. https://www.mkgandhi.org/ebks/ moralbasis_vegetarianism.pdf

18. https://www.choosemyplate.gov/resources/MyPlatePlan

19. https://www.nin.res.in/downloads/ DietaryGuidelinesforNINwebsite.pdf

20. https://www.who.int/nutrition/topics/ageing/en/index1.html

21. http://www.bmhegde.com/ideal_food.htm

22. https://www.havyakafoods.com/p/about-blog.html

23. https://airiefvision.wordpress.com/2020/10/29/health-wellness-keep-your-legs-strong/

24. https://veinatlanta.com/your-second-heart/

25. Unknown sources from social media

26. http://shaneomara.com/in-praise-of-walking
27. https://www.nin.res.in/downloads/
    DietaryGuidelinesforNINwebsite.pdf

Chapter 11 The Spirit of Living

1. Unknown sources from social media
2. https://gerontology.wikia.org/wiki/
   List_of_the_verified_oldest_people
3. https://www.lonelyplanet.com/articles/okinawa-secrets-for-a-
   long-and-happy-life
4. https://www.telegraph.co.uk/health-fitness/body/secret-
   japanese-longevity/
5. http://www.bluezones.com
6. https://www.nytimes.com/2017/07/25/science/shigheaki-
   hinohara-dead-doctor-promoted-longevity-in-japan.html
7. http://www.openculture.com/2017/08/10-longevity-tips-
   from-dr-shigeaki-hinohara-japans-105-year-old-longevity-
   expert.html

CPSIA information can be obtained
at www.ICGtesting.com
Printed in the USA
BVHW071141131221
623918BV00006B/94